HEALED ALREADY: IT IS FINISHED!

Receiving What the Cross Has Completed!

Gerard Assey

HEALED ALREADY: IT IS FINISHED!

Receiving What the Cross Has Completed!

By

Gerard Assey

Published by:
Gerard Assey
19/18, Palli Arasan Street
Anna Nagar East
Chennai - 600 102

ISBN: 978-81-995134-9-5

Table of Contents

This book is dedicated to the
Finished Work of the Cross*-*
and to my beloved
Wife, June,
with whom I have walked for
forty years (as of 2025),
and for whom JESUS has
already completed the work of
healing.
Thank you JESUS!

Dedication & Personal Testimony

Why This Book Was Written

This book is written as a dedication to the finished work of the Cross—and to my wife, June, with whom I have walked for forty years. It is not written out of fear, desperation, or unanswered questions. It is written out of conviction. A conviction forged not in a classroom, but in a hospital corridor. Not in theory, but in lived reality.

During the first week of December, something changed abruptly.

June, who had always been energetic and dependable, suddenly began feeling unusually giddy. Her appetite vanished almost overnight. Anyone who knows her would understand how concerning this was—she had always been strong, involved, and tirelessly active. Though she had experienced high blood pressure many years earlier, it had stabilized, and medication had been discontinued as she felt that there was no need. She also lived with arthritis, largely due to years of standing as a teacher, compounded by being overweight. For this, she had taken various Indian and herbal medicines over a long period.

Apart from these manageable concerns, she was otherwise well. In fact, she carried much of the home on her shoulders while I worked long hours. She was deeply involved in a Christian women's intercessory group, praying faithfully for the health and needs of others. She also devoted herself to our four grandchildren, tutoring them daily after school and pouring into their lives with patience and love.

Nothing about her suggested fragility.

One evening, as was my routine, I came home for tea around 4:30 pm before returning to my office downstairs. That day, she said something she had never said before.

“Love, don’t leave me and go down.”

Those words stopped me.

June had always been brave and independent. She rarely asked for help and never for reassurance. Something in her voice told me this was not an emotional request—it was a signal. I immediately insisted that we go to the doctor. She tried to reassure me, saying everything would be fine and that there was nothing to worry about. But I knew better. This was not imagination. Something was seriously wrong.

We rushed to the nearest clinic, where her blood pressure was checked. The reading was 236.

The doctor’s response was immediate and urgent. This level was extremely life-threatening. Medication was administered without delay, and by the grace of God, her blood pressure normalized within two days.

But the crisis was not over.

She continued to feel weak and giddy. Her appetite did not return. Whatever little food she attempted to take was vomited. This persistent condition alarmed us, and further investigations were ordered. Tests on her vital organs revealed something far more serious—her kidneys had been severely affected.

We were advised to move her immediately to Kauvery Hospital.

There, dialysis was initiated without delay. The doctors explained that the damage was most likely the result of prolonged hypertension combined with long-term use of non-allopathic medications for arthritis. The explanation was clinical, measured, and honest. There was no drama—just facts.

June is continuing treatment and will do so from home as well.

But this book is not written because of what doctors said.

It is written because of what Jesus already said.

At no point did I believe that heaven was scrambling for answers. At no point did I believe that God was "deciding" whether to heal my wife. I did not believe that this moment caught Him off guard. The Cross had already spoken long before December arrived.

I know that June is well—not because I deny medical realities, but because I trust a greater finished reality. Jesus has already completed the work for her on Calvary. Healing was not postponed, negotiated, or conditional. It was accomplished.

What is unfolding now is not God beginning a work—it is the physical manifestation of a work already finished.

This book was written so that others would not have to live beneath what Christ has already provided. It is written so believers can rest in truth, not wrestle with uncertainty. It is written to anchor faith—not hype it, not pressure it, not weaponize it.

Above all, it is written to honor Jesus.

And it is written with deep gratitude—for my wife, June, whose life continues to testify that the Cross did not fail, does not fail, and will never fail.

Preface

How This Book Is Meant to Be Read

This book was not written to convince God to heal anyone.

It was written to help believers understand what God has already done.

Healing is one of the most tender subjects in the Christian life because it sits at the intersection of faith, suffering, hope, and unanswered questions. Many sincere believers carry deep love for God while quietly wondering why healing seems elusive. Others have been wounded by teachings that felt heavy, accusatory, or dismissive of real pain.

This book was not written from that spirit.

It does not deny medical wisdom, dismiss ongoing treatment, or shame those who are still believing. It does not suggest that suffering is simple or that faith is effortless. It does not promise instant results or offer formulas.

Instead, it gently but firmly anchors the reader in one unchanging truth: the work of redemption, including healing, was completed at the Cross.

Every chapter flows from that foundation.

This book is meant to be read slowly. It is not a manual to rush through, but a truth to settle into. Some readers may need to pause often, reflect, or even revisit certain chapters more than once. That is not failure—it is wisdom.

If you are suffering as you read this, know this: you are not being evaluated. You are being invited. Faith is not forced, and healing is not earned. Nothing in this book requires you to pretend, deny symptoms, or silence questions.

You will notice that the emphasis throughout is not on trying harder, praying louder, or believing better—but on resting deeper in what Jesus has already finished.

The Cross does not need assistance. It needs understanding.

My prayer is that as you read, fear will lose its voice, condemnation will loosen its grip, and faith will rise—not as pressure, but as peace.

Read with an open heart. Let truth do the work.

INTRODUCTION
Living From a Finished Reality

Most believers are sincere. Many are devoted. Yet far too many are still striving for what Christ already completed.

This book was written because there is a silent struggle in the Body of Christ—one that often goes unnoticed and unaddressed. It is the struggle of believers who love God deeply, yet live as though redemption is still *in progress* rather than *complete*. They pray for healing as though it must still be earned, contend for victory as though it is uncertain, and battle condemnation as though the cross merely made forgiveness possible, not final.

At the heart of this struggle lies a single misunderstanding: We know the cross happened—but we do not fully live from what it finished.

When Jesus cried, *"Tetelestai"—"It is finished"*—He was not making an emotional statement in His final moments. He was issuing a legal, spiritual, and eternal declaration. In that one word, the debt of sin was cancelled, the curse was broken, sickness was judged, separation was ended, and the believer's new reality was sealed forever.

Yet today, many Christians still live as though the work of the cross is partial—powerful, yes, but incomplete; sufficient in theory, yet insufficient in daily experience. We are often taught how to ask God to do what Scripture says Christ has already done.

This book does not present a new doctrine. It restores an ancient truth.
It calls the believer back to the center of the Gospel—not effort, not performance, not religious striving—but the finished work of the cross.
Healed Already: It Is Finished! is not written to stir emotion alone, but to establish conviction. It is an invitation to shift from a mindset of waiting to one of receiving, from pleading to believing, from fighting for victory to enforcing it.
These pages will take you on a journey through:

- ✓ *The meaning of Tetelestai beyond the English phrase "It is finished"*
- ✓ *What the cross truly accomplished in the spirit, soul, and body*
- ✓ *Why many believers struggle to receive what is already theirs*
- ✓ *How faith responds—not by asking God to act, but by agreeing with what He has done*
- ✓ *How to live daily from a finished reality rather than a future hope*

This is not a book about denying pain or ignoring life's battles. It is about reframing them through the lens of the cross. When you understand what has already been settled in Christ, your prayers change, your posture changes, your authority changes, and your confidence before God is transformed.

The cross is not something we merely remember—it is something we live from.
As you read, do not rush. These truths are not meant to be skimmed, but received. Let Scripture speak. Let the Holy Spirit confirm. Let old assumptions be

challenged. And above all, let faith arise—not in what God *might* do, but in what He has *already done*.

This book begins where many teachings end— not at the struggle, but at the victory.

Because in Christ, the work is finished. And from that finished work, everything else flows.

Chapter 1
"Tetelestai" – The Cry That Changed Everything

There are moments in history that divide time itself—moments after which nothing can ever be the same again. One such moment occurred on a rugged hill called Golgotha, when a bruised, bleeding Savior drew His final breath and released a single word that thundered through eternity:

"It is finished." —John 19:30

At first glance, these words may appear to be the sigh of a dying man, the final utterance of someone who had reached the end of unbearable suffering. But nothing could be further from the truth. Jesus was not announcing defeat. He was proclaiming completion. He was not yielding to death; He was conquering it. This cry was not a whisper of weakness—it was a shout of victory.

The Greek word Jesus used was '***Tetelestai***'.

In the ancient world, *tetelestai* was written across legal documents and financial records when a debt had been fully paid. It meant *paid in full*, *completely satisfied*, *nothing more owed*. It was never used for something that was partially done or temporarily resolved. When *tetelestai* was declared, the matter was settled permanently.

When Jesus spoke this word from the Cross, He was declaring that the entire redemptive work He came to accomplish had been fully completed—sin atoned for, the curse broken, separation healed, and yes, sickness dealt with once and for all.

This is where many believers struggle, especially in the area of healing. We often think of healing as something God may do someday, if and when He decides the time is right. But Jesus did not say, *"It is beginning."* He did not say, *"It is now possible."* He said, *"It is finished."*

Healing was not initiated at the Cross. Healing was completed at the Cross.

Long before Jesus ever hung on that tree, the Holy Spirit had already revealed this truth through the prophet Isaiah. Writing more than seven hundred years earlier, Isaiah spoke of the Messiah in unmistakable terms:

"Surely He has borne our griefs and carried our sorrows… and by His stripes we are healed." — Isaiah 53:4–5

The words translated as *griefs* and *sorrows* are not merely emotional terms; they carry the meaning of sicknesses and pains. Isaiah was not describing poetic suffering alone—he was describing substitution. The Messiah would carry what did not belong to us so that we could walk free from it.

Peter, writing after the Cross, confirms this same truth, but with even greater clarity and finality:

"Who Himself bore our sins in His own body on the tree… by whose stripes you were healed."—1 Peter 2:24

Notice the tense. Peter does not say *you will be healed* or *you may be healed someday*. He says you were healed. The Holy Spirit is intentional with language. Past tense means the action is already complete. It points backward, not forward—to Calvary, not to the future.

This is where faith must shift.

Many sincere believers continue to pray for healing as though God is still deliberating, still deciding, still checking conditions. But Scripture reveals that the decision was already made—publicly, decisively, and eternally—when Jesus declared *tetelestai.*

Consider a believer Daniel. Daniel loved the Lord deeply. He was faithful in church, diligent in prayer, and sincere in his devotion. Yet for years he battled a chronic illness that drained his strength and clouded his joy. Every morning, Daniel prayed the same prayer: *"Lord, if it is Your will, please heal me. I trust Your timing."*

On the surface, this prayer sounded humble and reverent. But underneath it was a hidden assumption—that God had not yet decided.

One day, while reading the Gospel of John slowly and thoughtfully, Daniel paused at Jesus' words on the Cross. *"It is finished."* He sensed a quiet but firm question rise in his heart: *If it is finished, why am I asking God to start something He says is already done?*

As Daniel studied further, something shifted. He realized that he had been waiting for a future act of God, when God was inviting him to receive a finished work. His prayers began to change. Instead of pleading, he began thanking. Instead of waiting, he began believing. Instead of hoping, he began resting.

Daniel's body did not change overnight—but his heart did. Fear loosened its grip. Confusion gave way to confidence. And as his mind renewed itself in the truth of the Word, healing began to manifest where striving never could.

This is the power of understanding *tetelestai.*

Healing is not an optional add-on to salvation. It is woven into redemption itself. When Jesus bore sin, He also bore its consequences. When He took the curse, He addressed everything the curse produced—including sickness, disease, and brokenness.

God has never used sickness as a tool to teach His children. Scripture is clear about the source of healing and the source of affliction. The Lord declares, "I am the LORD who heals you" (Exodus 15:26), while Satan is consistently revealed as the oppressor and afflicter. Jesus Himself described His ministry this way:

"The Spirit of the Lord is upon Me…to heal the brokenhearted… to set at liberty those who are oppressed." —Luke 4:18

Oppression is never attributed to God.

If sickness glorified God, Jesus would have preserved it—not removed it. Yet everywhere He went, He healed **all** who came to Him. Never once did He say, *"This sickness is from My Father,"* or *"Remain ill for My glory."* His actions consistently revealed the Father's will.

The Cross, then, becomes the ultimate revelation of God's heart toward human suffering. Jesus did not negotiate healing there—He purchased it. He did not delay healing—He finished it.

This truth invites a necessary change in how believers speak and pray. There is a profound difference between asking God to do something and thanking Him for what He has already done. Gratitude is the language of faith because it acknowledges completion.

Instead of saying, *"God, please heal me,"* *the believer learns to say, "Lord, I thank You that by the stripes of Jesus, healing has already been provided for me."* This is not denial of symptoms; it is alignment with truth. Faith does not ignore reality—it chooses which reality has the final authority.

As the heart embraces this truth, daily confession becomes a powerful tool—not as a ritual, but as a renewal of the mind. Speaking Scripture such as 1 Peter 2:24 aloud anchors the soul in what Christ has accomplished. Over time, faith moves from theory to confidence, and confidence to rest.

The cry of *tetelestai* still echoes today. It calls believers out of striving and into trust, out of waiting and into receiving, out of uncertainty and into assurance.

- ✓ *Healing is not something God is withholding.*
- ✓ *Healing is not something heaven is delaying.*
- ✓ *Healing is not something the Cross failed to address.*
- ✓ *Healing was completed.*

And the invitation now is simple, yet profound:

Believe what Jesus finished—and learn to live from it.

Chapter 2
Jesus – The Perfect Picture of God's Will to Heal

One of the greatest struggles believers face when seeking healing is not pain itself, but uncertainty about God's will. The question that often whispers beneath prayers is not *"Can God heal?"* but *"Does He want to?"* Many sincere believers live suspended between hope and doubt because they have never fully settled this issue.

Scripture, however, does not leave us guessing.

God did not merely send messages to explain His will—He sent a Person. And that Person was Jesus Christ.

The writer of Hebrews captures this truth with breathtaking clarity: *"The Son is the radiance of God's glory and the exact representation of His being."* —Hebrews 1:3

The phrase *exact representation* is crucial. It means that Jesus is not a partial picture of God, nor a softened version suited for humanity. He is the precise imprint of the Father's nature. To see Jesus is to see God as He truly is—not filtered through tradition, fear, or human reasoning.

Jesus Himself affirmed this when He said: *"Anyone who has seen Me has seen the Father."* John 14:9

This statement alone dismantles countless misconceptions about God. If Jesus healed the sick, then healing reflects the Father's heart. If Jesus was moved with compassion toward the suffering, then compassion is not a temporary emotion—it is a divine attribute. If Jesus never refused a seeker, then refusal cannot be attributed to God's will.

When we read the Gospels carefully, a remarkable pattern emerges. People came to Jesus with every imaginable condition—leprosy, paralysis, blindness, hemorrhaging, fevers, demon oppression, and chronic infirmities. Some came boldly, others hesitantly. Some came with strong faith, others with fragile hope. Yet not once do we find Jesus turning someone away because it "wasn't the right time" or because suffering was *"working something good."*

There is no recorded moment where Jesus said, *"My Father wants you to remain sick for a season."*

There is no instance where He declared, *"This illness is for God's glory—keep it."*

There is no example of Jesus healing selectively while leaving others to wonder if God loved them less.

Instead, the Gospels repeatedly describe Jesus as being moved with compassion.

Matthew records one such moment:

"Jesus went out and saw a great multitude; and He was moved with compassion for them, and healed their sick." —Matthew 14:14

Compassion was not an accessory to Jesus' ministry—it was its driving force. Healing did not flow from obligation, performance, or merit. It flowed from the heart of God encountering human suffering.

To understand how radical this revelation was, we must look briefly at the Old Testament backdrop. Under the Old Covenant, God revealed Himself as Jehovah Rapha—The Lord Who Heals (Exodus 15:26). He healed bitter waters, preserved Israel's health in the wilderness, and restored individuals like Naaman the Syrian and Hezekiah the king. Yet much

of God's interaction with humanity was mediated through laws, priests, sacrifices, and prophets.
Healing existed—but it was often perceived as an act of divine intervention rather than a revelation of divine nature.
Jesus changed that.
In Christ, healing was no longer merely something God *did*—it became something God *revealed about Himself*. Jesus did not heal to prove His power; He healed to unveil His Father's heart.
Consider the leper in Mark 1 who approached Jesus with a question that echoes through generations:
"If You are willing, You can make me clean."
This man did not doubt Jesus' ability—he doubted His willingness. How did Jesus respond?
"Moved with compassion, Jesus stretched out His hand and touched him, and said, 'I am willing. Be cleansed.'"
Three words settled the matter: *"I am willing."*
In that moment, Jesus answered not just the leper's question, but humanity's. The will of God was no longer hidden behind mystery or theology—it stood before them, touching the untouchable.
Yet many believers today still struggle to reconcile this picture of Jesus with the beliefs they were taught growing up.
Consider a woman named Martha.
Martha was raised in a sincere Christian home where suffering was often spiritualized. She was taught that sickness builds character, that pain produces patience, and that healing should never be assumed. When she developed a long-term illness, well-meaning voices around her reminded her to "submit to God's will" and "learn what God is teaching."

But as Martha read the Gospels for herself, she became unsettled. She noticed something troubling: Jesus never taught people through sickness. He taught them through truth. He never corrected illness—He corrected minds and hearts. And wherever He found sickness, He removed it.

Martha found herself asking an honest question: *If sickness glorifies God, why did Jesus spend so much time undoing it?*

That question became a turning point.

Slowly, Martha realized that many of her beliefs about suffering were not formed by Scripture, but by tradition. She began to see Jesus not as a contradiction to God's will, but as its clearest expression. Healing was no longer something she hesitated to believe—it became something she expected because she finally understood who God is.

This is why Jesus must remain our interpretive lens for understanding God. Any belief about God that contradicts the life and ministry of Jesus must be reconsidered. If a doctrine paints God as distant, reluctant, or selective in healing, it does not align with the Jesus revealed in the Gospels.

Jesus did not heal people to advertise Himself. Often, He told them not to tell anyone. Healing was not a performance—it was a response. It flowed naturally from who He was.

When Philip once asked Jesus to show them the Father, Jesus responded with gentle astonishment: *"Have I been with you so long, and yet you have not known Me?"* In other words, *Look at Me. Watch how I live. Observe how I respond to suffering. That is what the Father is like.*

This understanding transforms how believers approach healing. Instead of asking, *"Is God willing?"* the question becomes, *"Will I trust what He has already revealed?"*

Studying the Gospels with this lens becomes a powerful exercise. As we observe each healing account, we are not merely reading history—we are discovering God's will in action. Every healed body becomes a declaration. Every restored life becomes a testimony. Every act of compassion becomes a mirror reflecting the heart of the Father.

And the revelation is unmistakable:

Jesus never refused healing—He revealed God's heart.

When believers begin to see Jesus clearly, faith no longer struggles against uncertainty. Healing ceases to be a theological debate and becomes a relational response. We trust God's will for healing not because of circumstances, but because we know His character.

Jesus is the will of God in flesh.

And in Him, that will was made unmistakably clear.

Chapter 3
Healing Is a Gift, Not a Reward

One of the most subtle yet destructive barriers to receiving healing is not unbelief in God's power, but misunderstanding God's grace. Many believers genuinely believe God *can* heal, yet quietly assume that healing must be earned, deserved, or qualified for. When healing does not manifest quickly, they turn inward—examining their failures, questioning their worthiness, and wondering what they have done wrong.

This mindset is not born out of rebellion; it is born out of religious conditioning.

From childhood, many of us were taught—explicitly or implicitly—that good behavior is rewarded and bad behavior is punished. While discipline has its place in parenting, when this model is projected onto God, it distorts His heart. God slowly becomes a taskmaster to be appeased rather than a Father to be trusted.

Scripture confronts this distortion head-on.

The apostle Paul writes with unmistakable clarity:

"For by grace you have been saved through faith, and that not of yourselves; it is the gift of God, not of works, lest anyone should boast." —Ephesians 2:8–9

Salvation, the greatest miracle of all, is a gift. It is not wages paid for good behavior, nor compensation for spiritual effort. No one qualifies for salvation through merit. It is received, not achieved.

Here is the crucial question this chapter asks: If salvation is a gift received by grace, why would healing—part of that same redemption—operate by a different system?

Paul anticipates this logic in his letter to the Romans:

"He who did not spare His own Son, but delivered Him up for us all, how shall He not with Him also freely give us all things?" —Romans 8:32

The word *freely* dismantles performance-based thinking. If God already gave His Son while humanity was still lost, broken, and sinful, then healing cannot be contingent upon moral perfection or spiritual performance. The Cross was not God's response to our worthiness; it was His answer to our need.

Healing, like forgiveness, flows from grace.

Yet many believers subconsciously treat healing as a reward system. They examine their prayer life, their fasting record, their consistency in church attendance, and their recent failures. When they find flaws—as everyone does—they conclude that now is not the right time to ask God for healing.

This is where guilt and condemnation quietly step in.

Condemnation does not always shout. Often, it whispers. It says things like, *"You should know better." "If you were more faithful, this wouldn't be happening."*

"God helped you before—don't ask again."

But condemnation never comes from God.

Paul declares boldly: *"There is therefore now no condemnation to those who are in Christ Jesus."* —Romans 8:1

Condemnation blocks faith not because God withdraws, but because the heart withdraws. When a believer feels unworthy, they hesitate to receive. They may still pray, but their prayers lack expectation. They may still quote Scripture, but their hearts remain guarded.

This is precisely what happened to a man we will call Samuel.

Samuel had walked closely with God for many years. But after a season of failure—choices he deeply regretted—he found himself battling a serious health issue. Though he knew the Scriptures, he delayed praying for healing. Each time the thought came, another followed quickly: *"Fix your spiritual life first."*

Samuel believed, without realizing it, that healing was something God might grant once he proved he had learned his lesson.

Weeks passed. His condition worsened. One evening, while reading Psalm 103, Samuel stopped mid-sentence:

"Bless the LORD, O my soul, and forget not all His benefits, who forgives all your iniquities, who heals all your diseases." —Psalm 103:2–3

The word *all* arrested him.

God did not forgive *some* sins and heal *some* diseases. The psalm tied forgiveness and healing together as benefits flowing from the same source—the mercy of God. Samuel realized something profound: if his forgiveness was secure despite his failure, then healing could not be withheld because of it.

That night, Samuel stopped striving and simply received. He thanked God—not because he felt worthy, but because God is good. In that posture of rest, faith finally found room to breathe.

This truth is not new. Even in the Old Testament, God repeatedly revealed Himself as gracious before He revealed Himself as powerful. When Israel murmured in the wilderness, God still healed their diseases. When Naaman the Syrian approached the prophet Elisha full of pride and misunderstanding, healing still flowed—not because Naaman behaved well, but because he obeyed a simple instruction rooted in grace.

Jesus reinforced this grace-based approach repeatedly in the New Testament.

He healed people before they had theology. He healed people before they corrected their lifestyles. He healed people who did not even return to thank Him. Healing was never portrayed as a medal for spiritual excellence. It was an expression of divine kindness.

This is why Jesus often healed first and addressed life change later. Grace opens hearts; law hardens them.

When believers view God as a Father, everything changes. A loving father does not withhold care from a sick child because the child made mistakes. He moves toward the child, not away. He does not demand performance before compassion; compassion motivates restoration.

Jesus revealed this Father-heart constantly. His parables portrayed a God who runs toward prodigals, feeds undeserving guests, and restores broken sons before they have the right words prepared.

Healing flows from that same heart.

To receive healing the same way one receives salvation is to let go of self-effort and trust in God's character. Salvation did not require emotional perfection, doctrinal mastery, or moral flawlessness—only faith. Healing is received the same way.

Rejecting self-blame becomes a necessary spiritual discipline. Not because accountability doesn't matter, but because the Cross already addressed sin fully. To carry guilt Christ has already borne is not humility—it is unbelief in the sufficiency of His sacrifice.

As believers learn to release performance-based thinking, faith becomes lighter, freer, and more confident. Healing is no longer pursued anxiously; it is received gratefully. Prayer shifts from striving to resting. The heart settles into the truth that God is not measuring us—He is loving us.

Healing is not a reward for the faithful few. It is a gift for the trusting many. And it flows not from our goodness—but from His grace.

Chapter 4
Is Sickness from God? Settling the Question Biblically

Few questions trouble sincere believers as deeply as this one: *Is my sickness from God?*

It is not a casual theological curiosity. It is a heart-level question, often asked in hospital rooms, whispered in prayer through tears, or silently wrestled with during long nights of pain. How we answer this question shapes how we pray, how we hope, and how we relate to God in our suffering.

Many well-meaning Christians, attempting to defend God's sovereignty, have unknowingly wounded faith by attributing sickness to Him. Statements like *"God gave this sickness to teach me,"* or *"This disease is His will,"* though often spoken with reverence, create a dangerous confusion. They blur the clear biblical distinction between the nature of God and the works of the enemy. Scripture never asks us to be vague about this matter. In fact, it goes to great lengths to draw a sharp line between the two.

To settle this question biblically, we must allow Scripture—not tradition, emotion, or experience—to define God's character and Satan's activity.

God Reveals Himself as Healer, Not Afflictor

The first time God formally introduces one of His redemptive names to Israel, it is not as Judge or Warrior, but as *Healer*. After delivering the Israelites from Egypt and purifying the bitter waters of Marah, the Lord declares:

"If you diligently heed the voice of the Lord your God… I will put none of the diseases on you which I have brought on the Egyptians. For I am the Lord who heals you." — Exodus 15:26

This is not poetic language. It is covenantal revelation. God is drawing a deliberate contrast: *the diseases of Egypt* versus *the health of those who walk with Him*. He does not say, *"I sometimes afflict and sometimes heal."* He says, *I will not put these diseases on you*. Then He anchors that promise in His identity—*I am the Lord who heals you* (Jehovah Rapha).

Healing is not something God occasionally does; it is something He is.

To claim that sickness originates from God is to contradict the very name by which He first chose to reveal Himself to His redeemed people. It would be like calling light darkness or calling truth a lie. God is not divided within Himself.

Satan's Role as the Afflictor: The Case of Job

Some point to the book of Job as evidence that sickness comes from God. Yet a careful reading reveals the opposite.

Scripture explicitly states:

"So Satan went out from the presence of the Lord and struck Job with painful boils from the sole of his foot to the crown of his head." — Job 2:7

The agent of affliction is named clearly—*Satan*. God does not strike Job. Satan does. God permits, but Satan executes. This distinction matters deeply.

Permission is not authorship.

A judge may allow a criminal trial to proceed, but the judge does not commit the crime. Likewise, God's sovereignty does not mean He is the source of evil.

Throughout Scripture, God permits human and spiritual free will, but He never becomes the author of destruction.

Job himself, in his anguish and limited revelation, says, *"The Lord gave, and the Lord has taken away."* But the narrator—the inspired voice of Scripture—has already clarified that Satan is the one doing the harming. This reminds us of an important truth: what suffering people say about God is not always accurate theology. Pain can distort perception, but Scripture corrects it.

If sickness were truly God's tool, Satan would not need permission to afflict—he would simply be unnecessary. Yet Scripture consistently portrays Satan as the one who steals, kills, and destroys, while God works to redeem, restore, and heal.

Jesus Settles the Matter Once and for All

If there were still any ambiguity, Jesus removes it completely.

"The thief does not come except to steal, and to kill, and to destroy. I have come that they may have life, and that they may have it more abundantly." — John 10:10

Jesus draws a clean, unmistakable contrast between two kingdoms and two agendas. Theft, death, and destruction belong to the thief. Life—abundant, overflowing life—belongs to Jesus.

Sickness steals strength, kills cells, and destroys bodies. By Jesus' own definition, it fits squarely within the thief's work, not God's.

Even more decisively, Peter summarizes Jesus' entire earthly ministry in one sentence:

"God anointed Jesus of Nazareth with the Holy Spirit and with power, who went about doing good and

healing all who were oppressed by the devil, for God was with Him." — Acts 10:38

This verse is profoundly clarifying. It does not say Jesus healed those oppressed by God. It says those *oppressed by the devil.* Sickness is described as oppression, and the source of that oppression is clearly identified.

Jesus never once told a sick person, *"Remain ill so you can learn submission,"* or *"This disease is my Father's will for you."* He healed lepers, restored blind eyes, straightened crippled limbs, and raised the dead. In doing so, He was not rebelling against the Father's will—He was revealing it.

Jesus is the exact representation of the Father's nature. To say God gives sickness is to accuse Jesus of undoing the Father's work everywhere He went.

Old Testament Shadows, New Testament Clarity

Some struggle because they see instances in the Old Testament where judgment and disease appear together. What must be understood is progressive revelation. The Old Testament reveals God truly, but not fully. Jesus reveals God completely.

Hebrews tells us that God, who spoke in various ways through the prophets, has now spoken fully through His Son. Where shadows existed, Jesus brings clarity. Where partial understanding prevailed, Jesus reveals the heart of the Father.

Even in the Old Testament, sickness is often connected to covenant violation, not divine cruelty. It is the *result* of separation, not the *desire* of God. And even then, God repeatedly reveals Himself as the One who heals when His people turn back to Him.

Healing is always restoration to God's original intent, never a deviation from it.

A Modern Story: The Damage of a Wrong Belief

Raghav, a sincere believer in his early forties, was diagnosed with a severe autoimmune condition. A well-meaning elder told him, *"God must be teaching you humility through this sickness. Don't fight it."* Raghav stopped praying for healing. He endured treatments with resignation rather than faith. His prayers became apologies instead of petitions.

Months later, while attending a Bible study, he heard Acts 10:38 explained clearly. For the first time, he saw sickness as an enemy Christ came to defeat, not a lesson God imposed. Something shifted. He began to pray differently—not demanding, but believing. Whether or not full physical healing came immediately, his spiritual posture changed. Hope returned. Fear loosened its grip. His relationship with God became warm again, not tense.

Wrong beliefs did not create his sickness—but they prolonged his bondage.

Settling the Question in the Heart

To say "God heals; Satan afflicts" is not simplistic theology—it is biblical clarity. This truth does not deny God's sovereignty, nor does it trivialize suffering. Instead, it preserves God's goodness while giving believers confidence to resist sickness without guilt or confusion.

God may use suffering redemptively, but He does not originate it maliciously. He brings light into darkness; He does not create darkness to teach us to value light.

When sickness comes, believers are not called to submit to it as God's will, but to submit to God while resisting the works of the devil. This was the pattern of Jesus. This is the model given to the Church.

Until this question is settled, faith remains conflicted. But once it is settled biblically, prayer becomes bold, hope becomes anchored, and God is seen not as the sender of affliction, but as the Father who longs to heal His children.

And that is the God Scripture consistently reveals.

Chapter 5
"Waiting on God" – A Misunderstood Concept

There are few phrases in Christian vocabulary that sound as spiritual—and yet cause as much quiet damage—as the phrase, *"I am waiting on God."* It is spoken with sincerity, humility, and often with genuine pain. Believers say it while waiting for healing, breakthrough, provision, or answers. On the surface, it appears noble. But when examined through the lens of Scripture, we discover that this phrase has been misunderstood, misapplied, and in many cases, has delayed people from receiving what God has already provided.

The core truth we must settle is this: in the matter of healing, you are not waiting on God—God is waiting on you to receive.

This statement does not minimize God's sovereignty or deny His timing in other areas of life. Rather, it clarifies a specific biblical reality: when something has already been accomplished through Christ, waiting is no longer faith—*receiving is.*

When Waiting Sounds Like Faith but Isn't

Jesus made a profound statement in Mark 11:24:

"Therefore I say unto you, *what things soever ye desire, when ye pray, believe that ye receive them, and ye shall have them.*"

Notice the order. Jesus does not say, "When you pray, believe that God will give them someday." He says, *believe that you receive them.* The believing happens at the moment of prayer, not at the moment of manifestation. Faith does not wait to feel better before believing; it believes before anything changes outwardly.

Many sincere believers have turned waiting into a substitute for faith. They pray, then wait—hoping that one day God will decide to act. But biblical faith prays, believes, receives, and then rests.

Hebrews 4:3 states, *"For we which have believed do enter into rest…"*

Rest is not inactivity; it is the confidence that the work is already done. Faith-rest means ceasing from striving, begging, and pleading—and instead standing on what God has already said and done.

Passive waiting, on the other hand, sounds spiritual but often hides uncertainty. It says, *"Maybe God will heal me. Maybe He won't. I'm waiting to see what He decides."* That mindset does not align with the revealed will of God concerning healing.

Healing Exists Now, Not Someday

One of the greatest misunderstandings about healing is the assumption that it must come down from heaven at some future moment. Scripture reveals something radically different.

Jesus taught us to pray in Matthew 6:10, *"Thy kingdom come. Thy will be done in earth, as it is in heaven."*

This prayer reveals that God's will already exists perfectly in heaven. Our role is not to convince God to change His will, but to receive and enforce His will on earth. And in heaven, there is no sickness, no disease, no pain, and no decay.

Healing is not being manufactured in heaven every time someone prays. It was secured once and for all at the cross. Isaiah 53:5 declares, *"By His stripes we are healed."*

Peter echoes this in the New Testament, writing, "By whose stripes ye were healed" (1 Peter 2:24).

The tense matters. ***Were healed***. Not *"will be healed when God decides."* Healing already exists in the spiritual realm, just as salvation does. The issue is not availability—it is reception.

When a sinner believes in Christ, they do not say, *"I'm waiting for God to save me someday."* They believe, receive, and then grow into what they have already received. Healing operates the same way.

Old Testament Insight: Israel at the Red Sea

We see this principle illustrated powerfully in the Old Testament. When Israel stood trapped between Pharaoh's army and the Red Sea, Moses cried out to God. God's response was surprising:

"Wherefore criest thou unto me? speak unto the children of Israel, that they go forward" (Exodus 14:15).

God had already given deliverance. The sea did not part while they waited—it parted when they moved in faith. Waiting would have meant death. Moving forward in trust activated what God had already purposed.

In the same way, many believers stand at the edge of healing, praying earnestly, crying sincerely, but remaining stationary—waiting for God to act—when God is saying, *"Go forward. Step into what I have already provided."*

New Testament Insight: The Healed Leper

In Luke 17, Jesus healed ten lepers. He told them to go and show themselves to the priests. Scripture says,

"And it came to pass, that, as they went, they were cleansed."

They were not cleansed while standing still. They were healed while obeying in faith—while moving forward before they saw evidence. Healing manifested *in motion*, not in waiting.

Faith does not demand proof before obedience. Faith acts because God has already spoken.

A Modern Story: Daniel's Long Wait

Daniel was a devoted believer in his early forties. Years earlier, he had been diagnosed with a chronic digestive condition that left him fatigued and uncomfortable almost daily. He prayed often and sincerely. Whenever anyone asked how he was doing, he would say, *"I'm waiting on God to heal me in His time."*

Daniel loved the Lord, attended church faithfully, and lived a morally upright life. But beneath his words was a quiet belief that God was withholding healing until some unknown condition was met.

One day, during a small Bible study, the leader gently asked him, *"Daniel, when did God decide to forgive your sins?"*

Daniel replied without hesitation, *"The moment I believed in Jesus."*

The leader then asked, *"And did you wait years to feel forgiven before believing you were forgiven?"*

That question unsettled him. Over the next weeks, Daniel began studying Scriptures about healing and redemption. He realized that he had been waiting for permission to receive what was already his inheritance.

Instead of saying, *"I'm waiting on God,"* he began saying, *"I thank You, Lord, that healing is mine because of Jesus."* His symptoms did not disappear overnight, but his posture changed immediately. Fear gave way to confidence. Striving gave way to rest. Within months, the condition that had dominated his life for years gradually lost its grip.

The turning point was not a dramatic prayer—it was the shift from waiting to receiving.

Why Heaven's Reality Matters on Earth

If there is no sickness in heaven—and Scripture clearly affirms this—then sickness has no eternal authority. It is not part of God's kingdom. Jesus never treated sickness as a mystery to be endured. He treated it as an enemy to be confronted.

Acts 10:38 says, *"God anointed Jesus of Nazareth with the Holy Ghost and with power: who went about doing good, and healing all that were oppressed of the devil..."*

Healing was not an exception in Jesus' ministry—it was the evidence that the kingdom of God had arrived. When believers say, *"Maybe God is using this sickness,"* they unknowingly attribute kingdom darkness to a kingdom of light.

Faith does not deny symptoms; it denies sickness the right to rule.

From Waiting to Receiving

The shift from waiting to receiving is not about forcing results. It is about aligning your heart with truth. Receiving says, *"Father, I trust You enough to believe You have already done what You promised."*

It thanks God before the body changes, before reports change, and before feelings change.

This is why thanksgiving is so powerful. Thanksgiving is faith speaking in the present tense. It is declaring agreement with heaven while still standing on earth.

When a believer moves from waiting to receiving, prayer changes. Worship changes. Language changes. And eventually, circumstances change.

God is not withholding healing to test your patience. He is not watching to see if you will wait long enough. He has already given His Son. As Romans 8:32 reminds us,

"He that spared not His own Son, but delivered Him up for us all, how shall He not with Him also freely give us all things?"

Healing is among those *"all things."*

The invitation of this chapter is simple but profound: stop waiting for what has already been given. Enter into faith-rest. Receive what grace has provided. And let heaven's finished work find expression in your body, here and now.

Chapter 6
Faith That Receives, Not Faith That Begs

One of the most subtle yet damaging misunderstandings in the Body of Christ is the confusion between *asking* and *receiving.* Many believers sincerely believe they are operating in faith, when in reality they are still trying to persuade God to do something He has already done. They pray passionately, fast earnestly, and plead repeatedly—yet deep within, there remains uncertainty about whether God is willing to act. This is not faith that receives; it is faith that begs.

The core truth of this chapter is simple but revolutionary: **faith is not persuasion—it is possession**.

Hebrews 11:1 defines faith with deliberate precision: *"Now faith is the substance of things hoped for, the evidence of things not seen."*

Faith is not a future wish; it is a present substance. It is not an emotional surge or mental optimism—it is the spiritual certainty that something already exists, even when it is not yet visible. Faith does not try to move God. Faith responds to God having already moved.

Faith Accesses What Already Exists

Biblical faith does not create realities; it *accesses* them. God is the Creator. Faith is the receiver. This distinction is vital. When believers pray as though healing must be generated through intensity or persistence, they unknowingly place themselves in the position of a persuader rather than a recipient.

Romans 4 gives us a profound insight into how faith operates through the example of Abraham. Scripture says that Abraham

"calleth those things which be not as though they were" (Romans 4:17).

This does not mean Abraham denied reality. It means he aligned his words with God's promise rather than his circumstances. His body was old. Sarah's womb was barren. Those facts existed. But God had spoken a greater truth, and Abraham chose to give voice to that truth instead of the limitations he could see.

The chapter goes on to say that Abraham did not waver in unbelief but was *"strong in faith, giving glory to God."* Notice that his strength in faith was expressed through glorifying God *before* the promise was fulfilled. He praised God not because the child had arrived, but because God had already spoken.

Healing faith operates the same way. It does not wait for symptoms to disappear before giving thanks. It gives thanks because God's Word has already declared healing accomplished.

Jesus and the Language of Possession

When Jesus taught about faith, He consistently framed it in the language of possession, not persuasion. In Mark 11:23–24, He said, *"Whosoever shall say unto this mountain, Be thou removed, and be thou cast into the sea; and shall not doubt in his heart, but shall believe that those things which he saith shall come to pass; he shall have whatsoever he saith."*

Jesus did not say, *"He shall have whatsoever he asks God to do."* He said, *"He shall have whatsoever he saith."* Speaking is not commanding God—it is aligning the heart and mouth with divine truth.
In the very next verse, Jesus adds, *"What things soever ye desire, when ye pray, believe that ye receive them, and ye shall have them."*
Receiving comes first in faith; having follows later in manifestation. Begging keeps the believer stuck in "someday." Receiving anchors the believer in "now."

Old Testament Picture: The Bronze Serpent
A powerful Old Testament picture of receiving faith is found in Numbers 21. When Israel was plagued by venomous snakes, God instructed Moses to lift a bronze serpent on a pole. Anyone who *looked* at it would live.
There was no begging involved. No pleading. No repeated sacrifices. Healing was not earned through effort—it was received through obedience and trust. Those who looked lived. Those who debated, delayed, or doubted died.
Jesus later revealed that this was a prophetic picture of Himself lifted on the cross (John 3:14–15). Just as healing flowed through looking then, it flows through believing now. The work has already been done. The response is faith.

Faith Speaks What the Heart Believes
One of the clearest indicators of whether faith is receiving or begging is language. Faith that begs says, *"Lord, please heal me, if it is Your will."* Faith that receives says, *"Father, I thank You that healing is mine through Jesus."*

Romans 10:17 tells us, *"So then faith cometh by hearing, and hearing by the word of God."*

Faith grows through exposure. What you hear repeatedly shapes what you believe deeply. And what you believe deeply will eventually be spoken—especially under pressure.

Speaking faith is not pretending symptoms don't exist. It is refusing to let symptoms have the final word. When believers continually rehearse pain, fear, and medical reports, they strengthen the voice of circumstance over the voice of truth. But when they speak Scripture—even with trembling—they are training their hearts to agree with God.

New Testament Example: The Woman with the Issue of Blood

The woman with the issue of blood in Mark 5 offers one of the clearest examples of receiving faith. Scripture says, *"For she said, If I may touch but his clothes, I shall be whole."*

Before she touched Jesus, before she felt healing in her body, she *said*. Her confession preceded her manifestation. She did not beg Jesus. She acted on what she believed. And Jesus responded not by saying, *"My power healed you,"* but, *"Daughter, thy faith hath made thee whole."*

Her faith did not persuade Jesus to heal her; it positioned her to receive what was already flowing from Him.

A Modern Story: Relearning How to Speak

Rachel had lived with recurring migraines for over a decade. She loved God and had prayed countless times for relief. Each episode drove her deeper into despair. Whenever pain came, her words followed a familiar pattern: *"Here it comes again. This never leaves. I don't know how much more I can take."*

She wasn't complaining—she was describing her experience. But over time, those descriptions became declarations.

During a Bible study on healing, Rachel encountered the idea that faith speaks truth before feelings change. At first, it felt unnatural—even uncomfortable. Speaking Scripture while in pain felt dishonest to her. But slowly, she realized she was not denying pain; she was denying pain authority.

The next time a migraine threatened, Rachel whispered through clenched teeth, *"By His stripes I was healed. My body responds to the Word of God."*

The pain did not vanish instantly. But something shifted internally. Fear lost its grip. Confidence replaced helplessness.

Over months, as she consistently spoke Scripture instead of symptoms, the frequency and intensity of the migraines diminished. What changed first was not her body—but her posture. Faith had moved from begging to receiving.

Why Faith Must Be Fed Daily

Faith is not sustained by memory; it is sustained by continual hearing. Just as the body needs daily nourishment, faith needs regular intake of the Word. When believers feed on news, diagnoses, and past disappointments more than on Scripture, faith weakens—not because God withdraws, but because attention shifts.

Daily declarations are not rituals; they are reinforcements. They remind the heart what is true when the senses argue otherwise. Over time, faith becomes less of an effort and more of a reflex.

Living from Possession, Not Petition

The invitation of this chapter is not to pray less, but to pray differently. Prayer rooted in faith does not sound desperate. It sounds confident. It thanks God for what has already been accomplished. It speaks to mountains instead of pleading about them.

Faith that begs remains uncertain. Faith that receives stands firm.

Healing does not come because faith is loud, emotional, or perfect. It comes because faith agrees with what Christ has already finished. When believers stop trying to convince God and start agreeing with Him, faith moves from striving to rest—and from hope to possession.

And that is the faith that receives.

Chapter 7
Renewing the Mind for Divine Health

Many believers genuinely love God, believe the Bible, and even agree—at least theologically—that healing belongs to them. Yet when sickness lingers, when symptoms return, or when medical reports worsen, something inside resists hope. That resistance rarely comes from the spirit. It almost always comes from the mind.

The mind is the most contested territory in the healing journey.

Scripture makes this unmistakably clear in Romans 12:2: *"And be not conformed to this world: but be ye transformed by the renewing of your mind..."*

Notice that transformation does not begin with a change of circumstances, but with a change of thinking. The word "renewing" implies that the mind does not naturally drift toward truth. It must be deliberately realigned—again and again—until it agrees with what God has already declared.

Why the Mind Resists Healing Truths

The human mind is shaped primarily by experience, repetition, and authority figures. From childhood, most of us have been trained to believe that sickness is normal, inevitable, and sometimes even permanent. We hear statements like *"This runs in our family," "You'll have to manage this for life,"* or *"At your age, this is expected."* Over time, these ideas sink deep, not as opinions but as assumptions.

When the Word of God introduces a higher truth—such as divine healing—the mind often reacts defensively. Not because the Word is untrue, but because it threatens what the mind has accepted as familiar and safe. Even pain can feel safer than uncertainty.

Proverbs 4:20–22 gives a remarkable insight into how God views His Word: *"My son, attend to my words… for they are life unto those that find them, and health to all their flesh."*

God does not describe His Word as symbolic encouragement or abstract theology. He calls it *life* and *medicine*. Yet like any medicine, it must be taken consistently—not sampled occasionally.

Old Testament Insight: The Twelve Spies and the Power of Perspective

A striking Old Testament example of the mind resisting divine promise is found in Numbers 13. Twelve spies were sent to survey the Promised Land. All twelve saw the same land. All twelve saw the same giants. But only two—Joshua and Caleb—processed what they saw through the lens of God's promise.

The other ten allowed past experiences of slavery and fear to shape their interpretation. They said, *"We were in our own sight as grasshoppers."* Their problem was not the giants—it was their self-image.

The Promised Land was already given by God. But an unrenewed mind kept an entire generation from entering what was already theirs.

In the same way, healing can be provided, promised, and purchased—yet still resisted internally by a mind trained to expect sickness.

How Long-Held Beliefs Delay Manifestation

Many delays in healing are not delays on God's side, but internal negotiations in the believer's mind.

Thoughts like *"What if this doesn't work for me?"* or *"I've believed before and nothing changed"* quietly undermine faith. These thoughts are rarely loud; they are subtle, familiar, and persistent.

Jesus addressed this inner resistance when He said in Mark 9:23, *"If thou canst believe, all things are possible to him that believeth."*

The father in that story responded honestly, *"Lord, I believe; help thou mine unbelief."* This was not hypocrisy—it was awareness. He recognized that belief and unbelief can coexist in the same heart, and that healing the mind is often part of healing the body.

New Testament Example: The Pool of Bethesda

In John 5, Jesus encountered a man who had been sick for thirty-eight years. When Jesus asked, "*Wilt thou be made whole?"* the man did not say yes. Instead, he explained why healing had not happened.

Years of disappointment had trained his mind to expect failure. Even standing before Jesus, he framed his future through past frustration.

Jesus did not argue with him. He simply commanded, *"Rise, take up thy bed, and walk."* Sometimes healing requires an interruption strong enough to override long-standing mental patterns.

A Modern Story: Learning to Think Differently

Samuel had lived with type 2 diabetes for over fifteen years. He managed it responsibly but had resigned himself to the belief that it would never change. Whenever he heard teachings on healing, he would quietly think, *"That's good for others—but not for me."*

During a season of intentional Scripture meditation, Samuel began reading Proverbs 4 daily. One morning, the phrase *"health to all their flesh"* struck him differently. He realized that his mind had never allowed "all" to include him.

He began a simple but disciplined practice: every morning and night, he read healing Scriptures aloud. When fearful thoughts arose, he did not argue with them emotionally; he answered them scripturally. Slowly, his internal dialogue shifted. Peace replaced anxiety. Expectation replaced resignation.

Months later, medical tests revealed significant improvement. But Samuel would tell anyone who asked: *"The biggest miracle happened before the numbers changed. My mind stopped resisting what God had already said."*

Word Intake as Spiritual Medicine

Just as the body requires consistent nutrition, the mind requires regular truth. Sporadic Scripture reading cannot undo years of fear-based thinking. Renewing the mind is not about intensity—it is about continuity.

When the Word becomes the dominant voice, fear loses its authority. Symptoms may still speak, but they no longer decide.

Isaiah 26:3 says, *"Thou wilt keep him in perfect peace, whose mind is stayed on thee."*

Peace is not the absence of symptoms; it is the presence of alignment.

Walking Daily in Mental Renewal

Renewing the mind for divine health is not a one-time event. It is a lifestyle. Each day presents a choice:

will the mind agree with the report of the body, or the report of the Lord?

Fear-based thoughts must be replaced intentionally, not ignored. Truth must be spoken until it becomes familiar, comfortable, and finally natural. Over time, what once felt forced becomes faith-filled.

Healing often manifests outwardly only after it has settled inwardly.

When the mind aligns with truth, the body finds permission to follow. And as the believer learns to think the way God thinks—about health, wholeness, and life—the finished work of Christ finds a clear path to expression.

This is not mental gymnastics. This is spiritual alignment.

And it is one of the most sacred steps in living healed already.

Chapter 8
Cooperating With the Finished Work

There is a moment every believer must come to—a quiet but powerful realization—that receiving healing is not about persuading God to act, but about aligning ourselves with what He has already done. The Cross was not partial, provisional, or symbolic. When Jesus said, *"It is finished,"* He was not announcing exhaustion; He was declaring completion. Healing, like forgiveness, was settled there once and for all.

Yet many sincere believers struggle at this very point. Not because they do not love God, or because they lack faith, but because they do not yet understand how to cooperate with the finished work. This chapter is not about striving harder, praying louder, or trying to qualify for healing. It is about learning how to receive what grace has already provided.

Everything begins with the nature of God.

Before faith can rest, the heart must be settled about who God is. Scripture reveals Him unmistakably as a good Father. From the opening pages of Genesis, we see that everything He created was declared "good." There is no sickness in His design, no disease in His intent, no harm in His heart toward His children. Jesus reinforced this truth when He asked, *"Which of you, if your son asks for bread, will give him a stone?"* The question answers itself. A loving father does not wound his child to teach him a lesson.

Yet many believers, often without realizing it, carry a distorted view of God when sickness enters their lives. Statements such as *"God wanted this,"* or *"God is teaching me something through this illness,"* may sound humble, but they quietly erode faith. If sickness were truly God's will, then seeking healing would be resistance to His purpose. If disease were divine instruction, then doctors would be interrupting God's curriculum. Jesus never taught this way, nor did He model it.

Throughout the Gospels, Jesus healed freely, fully, and without discrimination. He never turned anyone away saying, "*This sickness is from My Father,"* or "*This suffering is necessary for your growth."* Acts 10:38 summarizes His ministry plainly: He went about doing good and healing all who were oppressed by the devil. Healing was consistently presented as good, and oppression as evil. This distinction matters deeply, because faith cannot grow where God's character is confused.

Once the goodness of God is settled, the next clarity Scripture brings is equally important: God is not the author of sickness. Oppression has a source, and it is not heaven. Jesus Himself identified the thief as the one who steals, kills, and destroys, while declaring that He came to give life in abundance. There is a clear division between the life-giving nature of God and the destructive work of the enemy. This understanding removes fear and blame. God does not punish His children with disease. Correction, discipline, and conviction may come from the Lord, but sickness is never listed among the tools of a loving Father. Recognizing this truth restores confidence. It allows a believer to resist sickness without feeling rebellious or irreverent.

James writes that when the devil is resisted, he flees. Resistance implies authority, and authority implies position. In Christ, believers are not victims pleading for relief; they are children standing on legal ground. Even Jesus, when tempted in the wilderness, did not argue emotionally with the enemy. He simply wielded the Word. Scripture silenced deception then, and it still does now.

Many believers also struggle under the weight of supposed curses—spoken words, generational patterns, or fearful diagnoses that feel bigger than faith. Scripture addresses this directly. Galatians 3:13 declares that Christ has redeemed us from the curse of the law by becoming a curse for us. Every curse listed under the law, including sickness and disease, was placed upon Him. Redemption is not partial. There is no remaining category of "special curses" left uncovered by the Cross.

This means the believer does not need to search endlessly for hidden causes before receiving healing. The Cross already dealt with the root. Faith does not begin with fear of curses; it begins with confidence in redemption.

At the heart of this entire journey stands one unshakable truth: healing is already finished. *"By His stripes we were healed,"* Peter writes—not "we will be," but "we were." The tense matters. Scripture places healing in the completed work of Christ, not in the believer's future effort.

Salvation itself reveals this pattern. The Greek word *sozo* includes forgiveness, healing, deliverance, and restoration. When a person is saved, they do not receive forgiveness immediately and wait years for redemption to become valid. Forgiveness was accomplished at the Cross and received by faith. Healing operates under the same covenant.

A helpful way to understand this is to think of a bank account. A person may desperately need money, yet have a fully funded account they are unaware of. The issue is not provision, but access. Healing already exists in the spiritual realm because Jesus paid for it. Faith does not create healing; it withdraws what already belongs to the believer.

This is why waiting passively for “God’s time” can unintentionally dishonor the finished work. Many have waited in despair for something that was already provided, simply because they did not know how to receive it.

God’s chosen delivery system for healing is His Word. Scripture tells us that He sent His Word and healed them. The Word of God is not merely informational; it is active, living, and powerful. Isaiah records that God’s Word never returns void—it accomplishes what He sends it to do. Healing is one of those divine assignments.

When the centurion approached Jesus on behalf of his servant, he did not ask for a physical visit. He understood authority. “Speak the word only,” he said, “and my servant will be healed.” Jesus marveled at this faith. At that very moment, the healing command was released, and the servant was restored. Distance was irrelevant. The Word traveled instantly.

The writer of Hebrews explains that the Word penetrates even to dividing soul and spirit, joints and marrow. Healing often flows first into the unseen places—beliefs, thoughts, expectations—before manifesting in the body. This is why renewing the mind is not optional. It is part of the healing process.

Still, sincere believers often ask, “If God’s will is healing, why isn’t everyone healed?” Scripture answers this question gently, without blame. God desires all to be saved, yet not all are saved. Desire does not override human response. Healing, like salvation, involves cooperation.

There are multiple factors that can affect manifestation. Sometimes it is simple ignorance—not knowing what Christ has already done. Hosea writes that God’s people are destroyed for lack of knowledge, not lack of love. Other times it is unbelief, often rooted in past disappointment or conflicting teaching. Even Jesus encountered this limitation in His hometown, where Scripture says He could do no mighty works because of their unbelief.

Self-pity, fear, or unresolved inner wounds can also cloud expectation. None of these disqualify a believer from God’s love, but they can hinder reception. The enemy, too, works through deception, attempting to magnify symptoms and silence truth. And occasionally, the unbelief of others creates an atmosphere of doubt that must be intentionally resisted.

The solution is not condemnation, but light. Healing flows where truth is welcomed.

Jesus also taught His disciples not merely to pray about problems, but to speak to them. Faith is not always expressed upward; sometimes it must be directed outward. When Jesus spoke of commanding the mountain to move, He was teaching authority-based faith. The believer is not asking the mountain politely; they are exercising delegated authority.

This is why Scripture encourages believers to address sickness directly, in the name of Jesus. Disease has a name, but His name is above every name. At the name of Jesus, every knee must bow—whether in heaven, on earth, or under the earth. That includes the names given to sickness and pain.

Healing in Scripture is never limited to symptom removal. Jesus consistently healed the whole person. When the woman with the issue of blood reached out in faith, she did not merely receive physical relief; Jesus declared her whole. Wholeness includes peace, restoration, dignity, and freedom from fear. Healing is not meant to return a person to survival mode, but to restore them to life.

Faith must also be released. Possessing faith and expressing faith are not the same. Throughout Scripture, God often used points of contact—not because they carried power, but because they helped people release faith. A touch, a step, a lifted hand, obedience to a simple instruction—these moments became turning points. Faith without expression remains dormant.

Spiritual practices such as praying in the Spirit, partaking in Communion, and living a life of praise further strengthen and sustain health. These are not formulas, but invitations into ongoing fellowship with God. Praise, in particular, protects what faith has received. Thanksgiving anchors the heart in truth and keeps the soul aligned with heaven's perspective.

Ultimately, healing is not meant to make a believer inward-focused. It is meant to release them into purpose. Paul survived shipwreck not because the storm was small, but because the call on his life was not yet fulfilled. Purpose strengthens perseverance. Testimony multiplies hope. When believers share God's goodness, faith grows—not only in others, but in their own hearts.

God does not require His children to live dependent on another person's faith forever. While receiving prayer from others is a blessing, every believer is called to grow into personal confidence in Christ's finished work. Healing, like salvation, is meant to be lived from—not visited occasionally.

There is no sickness in heaven. When Jesus taught us to pray, "Your will be done on earth as it is in heaven," He was inviting us to align earthly experience with heavenly reality. Healing is not foreign to God's kingdom. It is native there.

The Cross has already spoken. Heaven is already settled. Learning to cooperate with the finished work is simply learning to agree—with faith, with humility, and with trust.

And agreement is where manifestation begins.

Chapter 9
Standing in Faith While Symptoms Persist

One of the most misunderstood—and emotionally challenging—parts of the healing journey is what to do when faith has been exercised, prayers have been prayed, Scripture has been spoken, yet symptoms remain. This is the space where confusion creeps in, where faith is tested not by intensity but by endurance, and where many believers mistakenly conclude that they have failed God—or worse, that God has failed them.

But symptoms do not cancel truth.

The Apostle Paul captures the posture of faith in a single sentence: *"For we walk by faith, not by sight"* (2 Corinthians 5:7).

Walking by faith does not mean pretending we cannot see what is happening in our bodies. It means refusing to let what is seen override what God has said. Faith is not blindness; it is allegiance.

Faith Versus Denial

One of the most damaging errors in healing teaching is the idea that acknowledging symptoms equals unbelief. This misunderstanding has caused unnecessary guilt and emotional pressure for many sincere believers. Denial says, *"Nothing is wrong."* Faith says, *"Something may be wrong, but it does not have the final word."*

Even Jesus acknowledged reality before releasing power. When He encountered the blind, the lame, and the sick, He did not ignore their condition. He addressed it—and then transformed it.

In John 11, when Lazarus died, Jesus did not deny death. He wept. Yet He also declared, *"This sickness is not unto death, but for the glory of God."* Jesus held compassion and authority together. Faith does the same.

Standing in faith while symptoms persist is not about forcing smiles or silencing pain. It is about anchoring the heart in truth while walking through an unfolding process.

Old Testament Example: Job's Tension Between Pain and Trust

The book of Job presents one of the clearest biblical pictures of perseverance amid unresolved suffering. Job experienced severe physical affliction, emotional anguish, and relational isolation. He voiced his pain honestly. He questioned. He lamented.

Yet in the midst of it all, he declared,

"Though he slay me, yet will I trust in him" (Job 13:15).

Job's statement was not a declaration of God's cruelty, but of unwavering trust. He did not understand the "why," but he refused to let go of the "who." His perseverance was not passive resignation; it was stubborn confidence in God's character.

James later reflects on Job's journey, saying, *"Ye have heard of the patience of Job, and have seen the end of the Lord; that the Lord is very pitiful, and of tender mercy"* (James 5:11).

The "end of the Lord" reveals God's heart—not affliction, but restoration.

Perseverance Without Pressure
James 1:3–4 tells us that *"the trying of your faith worketh patience. But let patience have her perfect work…"*
Patience here is not waiting in frustration. It is steadfastness—remaining anchored when circumstances fluctuate. Perseverance becomes harmful only when it is fueled by pressure instead of peace.
Some believers unknowingly turn perseverance into performance. They feel they must "hold on harder," speak louder, or prove their faith through strain. But biblical perseverance is not anxious striving. It is quiet consistency.
Faith rests even while it stands.

New Testament Example: Paul's Thorn and Grace in the Process
In 2 Corinthians 12, Paul speaks of a "thorn in the flesh" that caused him great distress. He prayed three times for its removal, yet God responded with these words:
"My grace is sufficient for thee: for my strength is made perfect in weakness."
This passage has often been misunderstood as God refusing healing. But what is undeniable is that God did not condemn Paul for asking, nor did He withdraw His presence. Grace sustained Paul in the process.
The lesson here is not that believers should accept sickness, but that God's love does not waver during seasons of unresolved tension. Faith can coexist with unanswered questions without becoming fractured.

A Modern Story: Faith With Wisdom

Anita was diagnosed with an autoimmune condition that affected her mobility. She believed in divine healing and prayed fervently. At the same time, she followed medical advice and underwent treatment. Some around her accused her of lacking faith. Others told her to stop praying and "accept reality."

She chose a third path—the path of wisdom.

Anita continued to declare God's promises daily. She thanked God for healing even on days when movement was painful. She also took her medication faithfully, seeing it not as a contradiction to faith, but as a tool of God's common grace.

Over time, her condition stabilized and gradually improved. But more importantly, Anita remained free from condemnation. She did not measure her faith by symptom changes alone, but by her trust in God's character.

Her journey revealed an important truth: faith is not threatened by wisdom, and wisdom does not negate faith.

Trusting God Without Condemnation

Romans 8:1 declares, "There is therefore now no condemnation to them which are in Christ Jesus."

Condemnation is never from God. When thoughts arise that say, *"You didn't believe enough,"* or *"You did something wrong,"* they must be recognized for what they are—accusations, not instruction.

Standing in faith includes standing against shame. God does not withhold healing to teach lessons through guilt. His corrections are gentle, and His guidance is rooted in love.

Choosing Hope Daily

Refusing discouragement is not an emotional decision—it is a spiritual discipline. Discouragement focuses on what has not changed. Faith focuses on who God is.

Each day, the believer chooses where to rest their gaze. Some days require courage simply to say, *"I trust You."* And that is enough.

Walking Faithfully, Not Fearfully

Standing in faith while symptoms persist does not mean standing alone. God walks with His children through every stage—whether immediate healing or gradual restoration. Faith is not measured by speed, but by trust.

Symptoms may speak loudly, but they do not speak eternally. Truth does.

And as the believer continues to walk—without denial, without pressure, and without condemnation—the finished work of Christ remains secure, active, and faithful.

Because faith does not crumble when sight disagrees. Faith stands.

Chapter 10
Authority, Not Fear – Enforcing the Finished Work

One of the great paradoxes in the Christian life is that many believers pray earnestly for things God has already given them authority to enforce. They ask repeatedly for intervention when Heaven has already issued a verdict. The Cross was not only a place of sacrifice; it was a place of transfer—where authority was reclaimed and handed back to redeemed humanity.

Healing is not enforced through fear, desperation, or volume. It is enforced through authority.

Jesus made this unmistakably clear when He said to His disciples,

"Behold, I give unto you power to tread on serpents and scorpions, and over all the power of the enemy: and nothing shall by any means hurt you" (Luke 10:19).

This was not a promise reserved for spiritual elites. It was a declaration of identity and position. Authority is not something believers grow into emotionally; it is something they step into by faith.

Understanding Believer's Authority

Authority is not the same as power. Power is ability; authority is legal right. A police officer stopping traffic does not rely on physical strength but on the authority vested in the uniform. In the same way, believers do not enforce healing because they feel strong, but because Christ has authorized them.

After His resurrection, Jesus declared, *"All power is given unto me in heaven and in earth"* (Matthew 28:18).

He then immediately delegated that authority to His followers. The Great Commission is not merely about preaching—it is about representing Heaven's rule on earth.

Mark 16:17–18 reinforces this truth: *"And these signs shall follow them that believe... they shall lay hands on the sick, and they shall recover."*

Notice the phrasing. It does not say "they shall beg God concerning the sick." It says *they shall lay hands*. This is action rooted in authority.

Old Testament Picture: Moses and the Rod

An early picture of delegated authority appears in Exodus when God asks Moses, *"What is that in thine hand?"* Moses replies, *"A rod."* That ordinary rod—once used for shepherding—became an instrument of divine authority.

Moses did not pray for the Red Sea to part. He stretched out his rod. He did not ask Pharaoh politely to release Israel. He spoke on God's behalf.

The authority was not in Moses himself, but in obedience to God's command. Likewise, authority over sickness is not about personal holiness or spiritual intensity. It is about alignment with God's Word.

Declaring Freedom Over the Body

Fear thrives where authority is unexercised. Many believers allow symptoms to dominate their thoughts, conversations, and decisions—not because they lack faith, but because they have not learned to speak *to* the condition instead of *about* it.

Jesus consistently addressed conditions directly. He rebuked fevers. He commanded paralysis to leave. He spoke to storms. He did not ask circumstances to improve; He instructed them to obey.

Authority-based prayer sounds different from fear-based prayer. It is calm, clear, and confident. It does not plead. It declares.

Romans 8:19 says that creation waits for the manifestation of the sons of God. The body itself responds when authority is exercised in faith.

New Testament Example: Peter at the Gate Beautiful

In Acts 3, Peter encounters a man who had been lame from birth. The man asks for alms. Peter does not pray a long prayer. He does not ask God to consider healing the man.

Instead, he says, *"In the name of Jesus Christ of Nazareth rise up and walk."*

This was not arrogance. It was obedience to delegated authority. Peter knew something crucial: healing had already been authorized through Jesus' finished work. His role was to enforce it.

The man did not gradually improve. He responded immediately to authority spoken in faith.

Resisting the Enemy Firmly

Scripture is clear that sickness is often linked to oppression. Acts 10:38 says Jesus went about *"healing all that were oppressed of the devil."* Healing, therefore, is not only a matter of restoration—it is a matter of resistance.

James 4:7 instructs believers to *"resist the devil, and he will flee from you."* Resistance is not passive endurance. It is active opposition.

Fear is one of the enemy's most effective tools. Fear weakens authority by shifting focus from Christ's victory to personal vulnerability. But 2 Timothy 1:7 reminds us, *"God hath not given us the spirit of fear; but of power, and of love, and of a sound mind."*
Fear must be addressed—not entertained. Authority grows when fear is confronted and dismissed.

A Modern Story: Learning to Speak With Authority
Michael had struggled with chronic respiratory issues since childhood. Every cold escalated into something severe. Though he believed God healed, his prayers were filled with anxiety. He often said, *"I just hope this doesn't get worse."*
During a teaching on authority, Michael realized he had been surrendering ground through fear-filled speech. The next time symptoms appeared, he did something different. Instead of panicking, he calmly spoke aloud: *"In the name of Jesus, I resist this. My body is healed by His stripes."*
The symptoms did not vanish instantly, but fear did. Over time, the episodes became less frequent and less severe. Michael discovered that authority does not require drama—only conviction.

Authority-Based Prayer in Practice
Authority-based prayer begins with recognizing position. The believer is seated with Christ in heavenly places (Ephesians 2:6). From that position, they speak downward into circumstances—not upward in desperation.
Such prayer is rooted in Scripture, spoken with assurance, and followed by thanksgiving. It is not loud. It is settled.

Living Free from Fear and Oppression

Enforcing the finished work of Christ means refusing to allow fear, symptoms, or past experiences to dictate identity. The believer does not fight for victory—they enforce victory.

Healing is not something to chase. It is something to guard and declare.

When authority replaces fear, peace settles in the heart. And where peace rules, the body often follows.

Because the Cross did not leave believers powerless. It crowned them with authority.

Chapter 11
Healing as a Lifestyle, Not an Event

For many believers, healing has been presented as a dramatic moment—an altar call, a powerful prayer, a sudden breakthrough. And while God certainly does heal in moments, His deeper desire has always been something more enduring: a life lived in wholeness.

Healing, in God's design, was never meant to be an occasional rescue. It was meant to be a way of living.

The apostle John captures God's heart with remarkable simplicity in 3 John 1:2: *"Beloved, I wish above all things that thou mayest prosper and be in health, even as thy soul prospereth."*

This verse reveals something foundational. God's desire for health is not isolated to the body alone. It flows in alignment with the soul and spirit. Divine health is holistic. It is sustained. It is relational.

Spirit, Soul, and Body in Alignment

Scripture consistently presents human beings as integrated—not fragmented. When one area is neglected, the others eventually feel the strain. Many believers pray fervently for physical healing while ignoring soul-wounds, chronic stress, unresolved fear, or spiritual exhaustion.

Proverbs 4:23 warns us, *"Keep thy heart with all diligence; for out of it are the issues of life."*

The word "issues" here refers to sources, boundaries, and flow. Life—health included—flows outward from the inner man. When peace is disrupted internally, the body often becomes the messenger.

This does not mean sickness is always caused by emotional issues. But it does mean that sustained health is often supported by inner alignment.

Old Testament Wisdom: God's Desire for Long Life

In the Old Testament, health was closely tied to obedience, rest, and trust. Proverbs 3:7–8 says, *"Fear the LORD, and depart from evil. It shall be health to thy navel, and marrow to thy bones."*

Notice the language. Obedience is not framed as religious obligation, but as nourishment. God's commands were never meant to restrict life—they were meant to preserve it.

The Sabbath itself was an act of healing wisdom. God commanded rest not because He needed it, but because humanity did. Chronic exhaustion was never part of Eden.

Jesus and the Rhythm of Rest

In the New Testament, Jesus modeled a lifestyle of wholeness, not urgency. Despite enormous demand, He regularly withdrew to quiet places to pray. He slept during storms. He refused to be hurried by crisis.

Jesus understood something modern believers often forget: sustained power requires sustained rest.

In Matthew 11:28, He invites us, *"Come unto me, all ye that labour and are heavy laden, and I will give you rest."*

Rest is not laziness. It is trust expressed physically.

Peace as a Preserver of Health

Isaiah 26:3 declares, *"Thou wilt keep him in perfect peace, whose mind is stayed on thee."*

Peace is not merely emotional comfort—it is spiritual protection. Anxiety, fear, and constant striving erode the body over time. Peace, on the other hand, acts like a guardrail.

Paul writes in Philippians 4 that the peace of God *"shall guard your hearts and minds."* Guarding implies defense. Peace protects.

Many believers chase healing while living in constant mental agitation. God invites them instead to a slower, steadier pace—where healing becomes natural rather than forced.

Stewardship of the Body

The body is not an enemy to overcome; it is a gift to steward. Scripture calls it the temple of the Holy Spirit (1 Corinthians 6:19). Temples are not abused—they are honored.

Stewardship includes practical wisdom: rest, nourishment, boundaries, and attentiveness. Faith does not reject responsibility. It embraces it.

God often works *through* wisdom, not apart from it.

A Modern Story: From Crisis to Continuity

Thomas experienced a powerful healing from severe gastric issues after prayer. For months, he rejoiced. But slowly, old patterns returned—overwork, irregular meals, constant stress. Symptoms resurfaced, not because healing was revoked, but because wholeness had not become a lifestyle.

Through counsel and Scripture, Thomas realized healing was an invitation, not a finish line. He began restructuring his days—prioritizing rest, Scripture meditation, and emotional boundaries.

Over time, his health stabilized—not just physically, but holistically. Healing became less about "fixing problems" and more about *maintaining alignment*.

Thanksgiving as a Way of Living

One of the most overlooked disciplines of divine health is thanksgiving. Gratitude shifts focus from what is lacking to what is already present. It reinforces faith without striving.

Paul instructs believers to give thanks "in all things," not because all things are good, but because thanksgiving keeps the heart anchored in trust.

Thanksgiving is faith at rest.

Living Whole, Not Just Healed

God's vision is not that His children move from sickness to sickness, crisis to crisis, miracle to miracle. His desire is that they live whole—spiritually grounded, emotionally settled, and physically strengthened.

Healing as an event may change a moment. Healing as a lifestyle changes a life.

As believers learn to walk daily in peace, obedience, rest, and gratitude, they find that health is no longer something they chase—it becomes something they carry.

Because the Cross did not merely purchase healing for emergencies. It opened the way for **divine wholeness**—every day.

Chapter 12
Testimony, Praise, and Sustaining Victory

Healing does not end with manifestation. In many ways, that is where stewardship begins. What faith receives, praise protects. What testimony declares, the enemy finds difficult to reclaim. God never intended healing to be a private victory kept silent in the heart; He designed it to become a living witness—strengthening the healed and awakening faith in others.

The psalmist David understood this well when he commanded his own soul: *"Bless the LORD, O my soul, and forget not all his benefits: who forgiveth all thine iniquities; who healeth all thy diseases"* (Psalm 103:2–3).

Notice that David speaks to himself. Praise here is intentional, not emotional. He chooses remembrance over forgetfulness, gratitude over distraction. Forgetting is often the first step toward losing ground. Praise keeps memory alive.

The Power of Testimony

Testimony is not self-promotion. It is truth-telling. The word "testimony" comes from the idea of bearing witness—declaring what God has done so that faith is multiplied.

Revelation 12:11 reveals a spiritual principle that reaches beyond persecution and applies directly to victory: *"And they overcame him by the blood of the Lamb, and by the word of their testimony."*

The blood of the Lamb secures victory legally. The word of testimony enforces it experientially. What Christ has accomplished must be spoken to remain active in daily life.

Testimony is not limited to dramatic stories. It includes ongoing acknowledgments of God's faithfulness—small, consistent declarations that reinforce truth.

Old Testament Pattern: Stones of Remembrance

In the Old Testament, God often instructed His people to mark victories physically. When Israel crossed the Jordan River, God commanded Joshua to set up twelve stones as a memorial. These stones were not for God—they were for the people.

Joshua explained that when future generations asked about the stones, the testimony would be told again.

Healing victories also need memorials—not necessarily stones, but spoken words, written reminders, and shared stories. These become anchors when challenges arise.

Praise as the Language of Faith

Praise is not a reaction to feelings; it is a declaration of allegiance. Faith speaks through praise because praise aligns the heart with truth.

Paul and Silas demonstrated this in Acts 16. Imprisoned, beaten, and unjustly accused, they chose praise in the darkest moment. Their praise did not ignore pain—it declared God's sovereignty above it. The result was deliverance not only for them, but for others who were listening.

Praise shifts the atmosphere because it shifts focus. It magnifies God rather than the problem.

New Testament Example: The Healed Leper

In Luke 17, ten lepers were healed as they went, but only one returned to give thanks. Jesus asked, *"Where are the nine?"* This was not disappointment—it was revelation. Gratitude completes the healing cycle.

The one who returned did more than say thank you. He positioned himself to receive deeper wholeness. Jesus said, "Thy faith hath made thee whole." Gratitude preserved what healing initiated.

Guarding the Healed Life

Healing, once received, must be guarded—not from God, but from fear, doubt, and forgetfulness. Old thoughts, past diagnoses, and previous patterns may attempt to reassert themselves. Testimony and praise act as spiritual sentinels.

When believers rehearse what God has done, they reinforce faith. When they speak only of past pain, they reopen doors to discouragement.

This is not denial—it is discernment.

A Modern Story: Strength Through Testimony

Lydia had been healed from severe arthritis after years of limitation. Initially, she kept the experience private, unsure how others might respond. Over time, fear returned—what if the pain came back?

During a small group meeting, Lydia felt prompted to share her story. As she spoke, faith rose—not only in others, but in herself. The testimony reminded her of God's faithfulness and reinforced her confidence.

From that day on, Lydia made testimony part of her lifestyle. She spoke openly of God's work, not as a boast, but as gratitude. The fear lost its grip.

Writing the Testimony in Faith

Writing one's healing testimony—even before full manifestation—is an act of faith. It anchors expectation and gives language to belief. It does not deny the process; it declares the promise.

Habakkuk was instructed to "write the vision." Writing makes faith tangible. It becomes a point of return when emotions waver.

Praise as a Daily Practice

Daily praise does not require perfect circumstances. It requires intention. Gratitude spoken daily trains the heart to remain aligned with truth.

Praise does not ignore reality—it reframes it.

Living as a Witness of Wholeness

God's desire is not that believers merely experience healing, but that they *become* witnesses of His goodness. Testimony and praise keep the victory alive—not as memory, but as momentum.

Healing is received by faith.

Victory is sustained by praise.

And testimony ensures that what God has done continues to bear fruit—both in the healed and in those who hear.

Because praise does not just celebrate the victory. It protects it.

Chapter 13
Keys to Receiving Your Healing
Receiving What the Cross Has Already Completed

1. Settle This First: God Is a Good God

The first and most important foundation for receiving healing is to be absolutely convinced that God is good—and that He does only good. Healing does not begin with faith for the body; it begins with faith in the nature of God.

From Genesis onward, Scripture records that everything God created was good. Sickness, disease, and death were never part of His original design. They entered the world through the fall, not through the Father's hand. A loving father does not harm his child to teach a lesson, and our heavenly Father is far more loving than the best earthly parent.

Yet many sincere believers have said, often through pain or disappointment, "God wanted me sick," or "It is God's will that I suffer." If that were truly the case, then seeking healing would be resisting God's will. One would logically refuse medical help, prayer, or treatment and simply allow sickness to take its course. But this reasoning collapses when held against Scripture and against the life of Jesus.

Jesus never made anyone sick. He never told a suffering person to endure illness for spiritual growth. He healed all who came to Him. Scripture records at least seventeen occasions where Jesus healed every sick person present, and many more where He healed individuals. He never refused healing to anyone.

He declared plainly, *"I have come that they may have life, and that they may have it more abundantly"* (John 10:10). The apostle John echoes this heart of God when he writes, *"Beloved, I wish above all things that you may prosper and be in health, even as your soul prospers"* (3 John 1:2). James reminds us that *every good and perfect gift comes from above* (James 1:17). Healing, therefore, flows from the goodness of God, not from suffering.

2. Understand the Real Source of Sickness

Once God's goodness is settled, the second truth must be clearly understood: God is not the author of oppression—Satan is.

Acts 10:38 tells us that Jesus went about *doing good and healing all who were oppressed by the devil*. Scripture makes a clear distinction between the life-giving nature of God and the destructive work of the enemy. Jesus Himself said that the thief comes only to steal, kill, and destroy, but He came to give life (John 10:10).

The primary weapon Satan uses is deception. He seeks to misrepresent God, distort truth, and convince believers that sickness is either unavoidable or divinely assigned. When deception is believed, authority is surrendered. But when truth is known, resistance becomes effective.

James 4:7 declares that when we resist the devil, he must flee. Resistance is not emotional shouting; it is standing firmly on truth. Jesus Himself demonstrated this in Matthew 4 when He resisted Satan using the Word of God. The sword of the Spirit, which is the Word of God (Ephesians 6:17), remains the believer's greatest weapon.

Isaiah 14 exposes the devil as far smaller than his reputation suggests. When seen in truth, he is not a giant to be feared but a defeated enemy to be resisted. He trembles at four things: the Word of God, the Name of Jesus, the Blood of Jesus, and genuine praise.

Scripture even declares that what the enemy has stolen must be restored. Proverbs 6:30–31 speaks of a sevenfold restoration. Many believers have never claimed back what was robbed through deception—including health. Yet God's justice includes restoration.

3. Know That Every Curse Has Already Been Broken

Some believers have been told that sickness is the result of a curse—spoken, generational, or unknown. While curses are real under the law, Scripture is clear that Christ has already redeemed believers from every curse.

Galatians 3:13 declares that Christ redeemed us from the curse of the law by becoming a curse for us. Every sickness listed in Deuteronomy 28—known and unknown—was part of that curse. Jesus bore it fully so that believers could walk in blessing, not bondage.

A believer does not need to fear curses, search endlessly for causes, or live under spiritual anxiety. The Cross has already dealt with it. Healing flows from redemption, not from striving.

4. Stand on the Finished Fact of Healing

First Peter 2:24 states, *"By His stripes you were healed."* The tense matters. It does not say *you will be healed* or *you are being healed*, but *you were healed*. Healing is presented as a completed act.

Salvation itself is a package. The Greek word *sozo* means to save, heal, deliver, and restore. Forgiveness of sins, healing of the body, and restoration of life are all included. When a person receives salvation, God does not partially redeem them; He fully restores what sin destroyed.

Many believers wait, saying, “It is not His time yet.” But waiting for what has already been finished is not humility—it is ignorance of the Cross. The work was completed over two thousand years ago. Healing exists already in the spiritual realm, just as money may exist in a bank account. Faith is not creating healing; it is withdrawing what already belongs to us.

5. Let the Word Do Its Work

God sent His Word and healed them (Psalm 107:20). His Word runs swiftly (Psalm 147:15). When God speaks, healing moves faster than natural processes. Isaiah assures us that the Word sent forth will not return void but will accomplish what it was sent to do (Isaiah 55:11). Healing is not slow in God’s economy. In Matthew 8:5–13, the centurion understood this truth, and Scripture records that the servant was healed *that very moment* when the word was spoken. The Word penetrates deeply, even dividing soul and spirit, joints and marrow (Hebrews 4:12). Healing reaches where medicine cannot reach.

6. Remove Hindrances to Receiving

If healing is God’s will, why do not all experience it? The same question could be asked about salvation. God desires all to be saved, yet not all receive. Reception depends on belief.

Several factors can hinder receiving: ignorance of what God has already done, unbelief, self-pity, fear, unconfessed sin, or wrong focus in prayer. God has already done His part. Healing does not happen *to* us without cooperation; it happens *through* faith.
Jesus Himself could do few miracles in His hometown because of unbelief (Matthew 13:58). Faith cooperates with God; unbelief resists Him.

7. Speak to the Condition, Not About It
Jesus taught His disciples to speak directly to problems. He did not tell them to beg God to act. In Mark 11:23, He instructed them to speak to the mountain and command it to move.
Healing authority has been given to believers. Instead of praying, "If it be Your will," we speak in faith, commanding sickness to leave in the Name of Jesus. This is not arrogance; it is obedience to delegated authority.

8. Exalt the Name Above Every Name
Every sickness has a name—but the Name of Jesus is above every name. Arthritis, cancer, infection, and disease must bow at His Name. Philippians 2:9–11 declares that every knee must bow and every tongue confess that Jesus Christ is Lord.
Healing responds to authority when exercised in faith.

9. Receive Wholeness, Not Partial Relief
Healing in Scripture is not partial or progressive by necessity—it is often immediate and complete. The woman with the issue of blood did not seek symptom relief; she said, *"I shall be whole."* Jesus responded by declaring her whole (Mark 5:28–34).

Faith believes now. Hebrews 11:1 says, *"Now faith is."* God will meet us where our faith is, but His best is completeness.

10. Release Faith Through a Point of Contact
Faith must be released. A point of contact is an act that triggers faith—laying on of hands, responding to an altar call, taking communion, or speaking a declaration.
The act has no power in itself, but it releases what already exists within. Faith without action remains dormant.

11. Strengthen the Body Spiritually
Praying in tongues strengthens the believer. Research has shown measurable immune system benefits when praying in the Spirit. Communion, too, is a powerful participation in Christ's healing life, as discussed elsewhere in this book.

12. Sustain Healing Through Praise, Purpose, and Testimony
Praise keeps faith alive. Gratitude shifts focus from symptoms to victory. Staying focused on God's call gives perspective, just as Paul remained anchored to his purpose even in a shipwreck.
Finally, testimony seals victory. Sharing God's goodness strengthens others and establishes healing in the heart.

There is no sickness in heaven. Jesus taught us to pray that God's will be done on earth as it is in heaven. Healing, therefore, is not a future hope—it is a present inheritance.

Chapter 14
DECLARATIONS OF HEALING
Receiving What the Cross Has Completed

How to Use This Chapter

These declarations are not prayers asking God to heal; they are faith proclamations based on what Christ has already finished (John 19:30).

- ✓ Read them aloud, slowly, and with faith (Romans 10:10).
- ✓ Personalize them by saying "I" or "my body".
- ✓ Repeat them daily, especially when symptoms speak louder than truth.
- ✓ The power is not in repetition, but in agreement with God's Word.

"My son, attend to My words… for they are life to those who find them, and health to all their flesh." — Proverbs 4:20–22

---

1. DECLARATIONS FOR AIDS / LIFE-THREATENING DISEASES

Scriptural Foundation:

Isaiah 53:1–6; Psalm 103:1–5; Psalm 91:9–16; Proverbs 4:20–27; Romans 4:16–21

Declarations

- ✓ I declare that Jesus bore this sickness in His body, therefore it has no legal right in mine (Isaiah 53:5).
- ✓ I proclaim that the Lord restores my life from destruction and renews my youth like the eagle's (Psalm 103:4–5).

- ✓ I will not die but live, and I will declare the works of the Lord (Psalm 118:17).
- ✓ My body responds to the Word of God, which is life and health to all my flesh (Proverbs 4:22).
- ✓ I walk in the covenant of divine protection—no plague comes near my dwelling (Psalm 91:10).
- ✓ Like Abraham, I am strong in faith, giving glory to God, fully persuaded that what He promised, He is able to perform (Romans 4:20–21).

---

2. DECLARATIONS FOR ARTHRITIS / BONE & JOINT ISSUES

Scriptural Foundation:
Psalm 34:20; Proverbs 3:7–8; Isaiah 40:29–31; Jeremiah 30:17; 1 Peter 2:24

Declarations

- ✓ I declare that the Lord heals me and restores my health (Jeremiah 30:17).
- ✓ My bones are preserved; not one bone is broken or decaying (Psalm 34:20).
- ✓ Strength is infused into my body—the Lord renews my strength (Isaiah 40:31).
- ✓ The Word of God is medicine to my flesh and strength to my bones (Proverbs 3:8).
- ✓ By the stripes of Jesus, my joints, bones, and cartilage are healed (1 Peter 2:24).

---

3. DECLARATIONS FOR ATTITUDE / INNER WELL-BEING

Scriptural Foundation:
Proverbs 14:30; 17:22; Psalms 128:1–6; 146:5–8

Declarations

- ✓ I declare that a sound heart is life to my body (Proverbs 14:30).
- ✓ The joy of the Lord is strength to my spirit and healing to my soul (Proverbs 17:22).
- ✓ My mind is aligned with truth; hope in the Lord fills me with peace (Psalm 146:5).
- ✓ I walk in the fear of the Lord, and well-being follows my life (Psalm 128:1–2).

---

4. DECLARATIONS FOR BLOOD-RELATED CONDITIONS

Scriptural Foundation:
Matthew 9:20–22; Leviticus 17:11; Psalm 107:20

Declarations

- ✓ I declare that the life of my flesh is in the blood, and my blood carries divine life (Leviticus 17:11).
- ✓ As the woman touched the hem of Jesus' garment, I receive healing now by faith (Matthew 9:22).
- ✓ My blood is purified, restored, and aligned with God's design.
- ✓ The Lord sends His Word and heals me, delivering me from destruction (Psalm 107:20).

---

5. DECLARATIONS FOR A BROKEN HEART

Scriptural Foundation:
Psalm 147:3; Isaiah 61:1–3; Luke 4:18

Declarations

- ✓ I declare that the Lord heals my broken heart and binds up my wounds (Psalm 147:3).
- ✓ Jesus has exchanged my mourning for joy and praise (Isaiah 61:3).
- ✓ I receive beauty for ashes and the oil of gladness instead of heaviness.
- ✓ My soul is restored; hope rises within me again.

---

6. DECLARATIONS FOR CANCER

Scriptural Foundation:
Isaiah 53:4–5; Psalm 91:16; Proverbs 4:22; Romans 4:17

Declarations

- ✓ I declare that every abnormal cell is subject to the authority of Christ.
- ✓ By the stripes of Jesus, my body is healed and restored (Isaiah 53:5).
- ✓ My body responds to the life-giving Word of God, not disease (Proverbs 4:22).
- ✓ I call my body whole, healthy, and restored, in Jesus' name (Romans 4:17).
- ✓ With long life, the Lord satisfies me and shows me His salvation (Psalm 91:16).

---

7. DECLARATIONS AGAINST DEMONIC ATTACKS

Scriptural Foundation:
Luke 10:19; Mark 16:17–18; Matthew 10:1

Declarations

- ✓ I declare that I have authority over all the power of the enemy (Luke 10:19).

- ✓ Every demonic oppression is broken—Jesus has set me free.
- ✓ I resist the devil, and he flees from me.
- ✓ My body and mind are under the lordship of Christ alone.

---

8. DECLARATIONS FOR DEPRESSION & EMOTIONAL DISTRESS

Scriptural Foundation:
Isaiah 61:1–3; Psalm 34:19; Proverbs 17:22

Declarations

- ✓ I declare that the Spirit of the Lord brings healing to my inner man.
- ✓ I receive the garment of praise instead of heaviness (Isaiah 61:3).
- ✓ Though afflictions may come, the Lord delivers me out of them all (Psalm 34:19).
- ✓ Joy rises within me; my heart is strengthened (Proverbs 17:22).

---

9. DECLARATIONS FOR EYESIGHT / VISION

Scriptural Foundation:
Isaiah 35:5; Matthew 9:29; Luke 4:18

Declarations

- ✓ I declare that the eyes of the blind are opened (Isaiah 35:5).
- ✓ According to my faith, let it be done unto me (Matthew 9:29).
- ✓ My eyes receive clarity, focus, and strength.
- ✓ Jesus has proclaimed recovery of sight, and I receive it now (Luke 4:18).

---

10. DECLARATIONS FOR FERTILITY & CHILDBIRTH

Scriptural Foundation:
Exodus 23:25–26; Psalm 128:3; Deuteronomy 7:14

Declarations

- ✓ I declare that there shall be no barrenness in my life (Deuteronomy 7:14).
- ✓ My body functions according to God's design and timing.
- ✓ The Lord blesses my womb and removes every hindrance (Exodus 23:26).
- ✓ Fruitfulness is my portion; I receive it by faith.

---

11. DECLARATIONS FOR FEVER

Scriptural Foundation:
Matthew 8:14–15; Luke 4:38–40; Acts 28:8–9; Psalm 107:20

Declarations

- ✓ I declare that Jesus rebukes fever, and it leaves my body immediately (Luke 4:39).
- ✓ Every abnormal temperature in my body aligns with God's design.
- ✓ As Peter's mother-in-law was raised and restored, I receive complete recovery now (Matthew 8:15).
- ✓ The Word of God enters my system and heals me from the root (Psalm 107:20).
- ✓ I rise from weakness into strength; this condition does not linger.

---

12. DECLARATIONS FOR FLU & INFECTIONS

Scriptural Foundation:
Exodus 15:26; Psalm 91:9–16; Deuteronomy 7:15; Acts 4:30

Declarations

- ✓ I declare that the Lord is my healer, and sickness has no authority over my body (Exodus 15:26).
- ✓ No epidemic, virus, or infection shall settle or multiply in me (Deuteronomy 7:15).
- ✓ My immune system is strengthened by the life of God.
- ✓ I dwell under the shadow of the Almighty; no plague comes near me (Psalm 91:10).
- ✓ My recovery is swift, complete, and without complications.

---

13. DECLARATIONS FOR HEARING PROBLEMS / DEAFNESS

Scriptural Foundation:
Isaiah 35:5; Mark 7:34–35; Luke 7:22; Exodus 4:11

Declarations

- ✓ I declare that the ears of the deaf are opened (Isaiah 35:5).
- ✓ Just as Jesus said, *"Ephphatha—be opened,"* I receive restored hearing now.
- ✓ Every blockage, nerve damage, or impairment dissolves under God's power.
- ✓ The One who created the ear restores its function perfectly (Exodus 4:11).
- ✓ I hear clearly, distinctly, and fully, to the glory of God.

---

14. DECLARATIONS FOR HEART CONDITIONS

Scriptural Foundation:
Proverbs 14:30; Psalm 73:26; Mark 5:34; Psalm 107:20

Declarations

- ✓ I declare that my heart is strengthened by the Lord (Psalm 73:26).
- ✓ Peace governs my heart; stress and fear lose their grip (Proverbs 14:30).
- ✓ My heart rhythm, valves, muscles, and arteries align with divine order.
- ✓ As Jesus said, *"Daughter/Son, your faith has made you whole,"* I receive wholeness now (Mark 5:34).
- ✓ Life flows freely through my body; no obstruction remains.

---

15. DECLARATIONS FOR MENTAL ILLNESS / PSYCHIATRIC DISTRESS

Scriptural Foundation:
Proverbs 17:22; Mark 9:25; Luke 10:19; Hebrews 12:12–13

Declarations

- ✓ I declare that my mind is healed and restored by the peace of God.
- ✓ Every tormenting thought, confusion, or oppression is silenced in Jesus' name.
- ✓ I have authority over every unclean influence affecting my mind (Luke 10:19).
- ✓ My thoughts align with truth, clarity, and soundness (Proverbs 17:22).
- ✓ Strength returns to my inner being; my mind is whole and stable.

16. DECLARATIONS FOR LEPROSY / SKIN CONDITIONS / INCURABLE DISEASES

Scriptural Foundation:
2 Kings 5:14; Matthew 8:2–3; Luke 17:15–19

Declarations

- ✓ I declare, *"Lord, You are willing,"* and I receive cleansing now (Matthew 8:3).
- ✓ As Naaman washed and was restored, my body is renewed completely.
- ✓ Every visible and invisible affliction disappears under God's power.
- ✓ My skin, tissues, and cells are restored to original health.
- ✓ I return to give thanks—I am healed, whole, and clean (Luke 17:19).

17. DECLARATIONS FOR LONG LIFE

Scriptural Foundation:
Psalm 91:16; Proverbs 3:1–2; 2 Kings 20:5–6; Deuteronomy 30:19–20

Declarations

- ✓ I declare that with long life the Lord satisfies me (Psalm 91:16).
- ✓ My days are prolonged in strength, peace, and purpose (Proverbs 3:2).
- ✓ Like Hezekiah, I receive added years ordained by God (2 Kings 20:6).
- ✓ I choose life, therefore I live to fulfill my calling (Deuteronomy 30:19).
- ✓ I flourish in old age, bearing fruit and remaining full of vitality (Psalm 92:14).

18. DECLARATIONS FOR OTHER INCURABLE DISEASES

Scriptural Foundation:
Isaiah 53:5; Psalm 103:2–5; Romans 4:16–21; John 4:50

Declarations

- ✓ I declare that no disease is incurable where the Cross has spoken.
- ✓ What doctors call irreversible, God calls subject to His Word.
- ✓ As Abraham believed against hope, I believe in the God who gives life to the dead (Romans 4:17).
- ✓ My body responds to the Word of God, not to medical verdicts alone.
- ✓ I receive restoration at the root—cells, systems, organs, and functions.
- ✓ The same God who raised the widow's son and added years to Hezekiah is active in my body now.
- ✓ I shall not die but live, and declare the works of the Lord (Psalm 118:17).

19. DECLARATIONS AGAINST PLAGUE, BACTERIAL INFECTIONS & VIRAL ATTACKS

Scriptural Foundation:
Exodus 15:26; Psalm 91:10; Acts 4:30; Deuteronomy 7:15

Declarations

- ✓ I declare that the Lord is my healer, and no plague has permission to remain in me.
- ✓ Every bacterial and viral agent is neutralized by divine life.

- ✓ My bloodstream, lungs, organs, and immune system are saturated with healing.
- ✓ No epidemic shall overpower the covering of the Most High (Psalm 91:10).
- ✓ As the apostles prayed and signs followed, healing flows now in Jesus' name.
- ✓ What entered my body unlawfully must exit completely.

---

20. DECLARATIONS FOR SKIN DISEASES & ITCHING CONDITIONS

Scriptural Foundation:
Matthew 8:3; 2 Kings 5:14; Luke 17:19

Declarations

- ✓ I declare, as the leper did, *"Lord, if You are willing,"*—and I hear Him say, "I am willing. Be clean."
- ✓ Every irritation, rash, lesion, and inflammation dries up and disappears.
- ✓ My skin is renewed, restored, and strengthened.
- ✓ As Naaman's flesh returned like that of a child, my skin is restored fully.
- ✓ I am not ashamed, hidden, or isolated—I am made whole.

---

21. DECLARATIONS FOR SPEECH IMPEDIMENTS & MUTENESS

Scriptural Foundation:
Isaiah 35:6; Exodus 4:11; Matthew 12:22

Declarations

- ✓ I declare that the tongue of the mute sings for joy (Isaiah 35:6).

- ✓ The God who made the mouth restores my speech clearly and fully.
- ✓ Every restriction, nerve impairment, or spiritual hindrance is removed.
- ✓ As Jesus healed the mute man, I receive clarity and freedom now.
- ✓ My voice will testify of the goodness of the Lord.

---

22. DECLARATIONS AFFIRMING THE WILL OF GOD TO HEAL

Scriptural Foundation:
Matthew 8:3; Psalm 107:20; Jeremiah 33:6; Mark 1:41

Declarations

- ✓ I declare that it is God's will to heal me—now.
- ✓ Jesus never said "no" to anyone who came to Him for healing.
- ✓ God does not afflict to teach; He heals to restore.
- ✓ I receive the revealed will of God, not confusion or doubt.
- ✓ Healing is not a special favor—it is part of redemption.
- ✓ The compassion of Jesus is active toward me today.

---

23. DECLARATIONS WHEN SOMEONE IS NEAR DEATH

Scriptural Foundation:
Psalm 118:17; Isaiah 53:5; 2 Kings 20:5; John 11:25

Declarations

- ✓ I declare that life belongs to God, not to death.

- ✓ The same Jesus who raised the dead is present here now.
- ✓ Strength returns where weakness has overtaken the body.
- ✓ The Word of God enters and revives every failing system.
- ✓ This person shall not die but live, according to God's purpose.
- ✓ Even now, nothing is too late for the Lord.
- ✓ I stand on the finished work of Christ—hope is not over.

---

24. DECLARATIONS FOR KIDNEY FAILURE / RENAL CONDITIONS

This section is written for those facing acute kidney failure, chronic kidney disease, dialysis, or any renal dysfunction—affirming that nothing is beyond the redemptive reach of the Cross.

Scriptural Foundation

Isaiah 53:5; Psalm 103:2–3; Jeremiah 30:17; Proverbs 4:20–22; Romans 8:11; John 4:50; Psalm 118:17

Declarations

- ✓ I declare that kidney failure is not my master.
- ✓ Jesus bore sickness in His body, and healing was completed at the Cross.
- ✓ By His stripes, my kidneys are healed—not in hope, but in truth.
- ✓ I speak life into my kidneys.
- ✓ I declare restoration of filtration, regulation, balance, and strength.
- ✓ Every nephron, every tissue, every system responds to the Word of God.

- ✓ I refuse to accept "irreversible" as the final word.
- ✓ The God who restored Hezekiah's life adds strength and time to me.
- ✓ Medical reports inform—but the Word of God decides.
- ✓ The Spirit who raised Jesus from the dead dwells in me now.
- ✓ That same Spirit releases resurrection life into my kidneys.
- ✓ What is weak is strengthened.
- ✓ What is damaged is renewed.
- ✓ What is failing is revived.
- ✓ If I am undergoing treatment, I declare this:
- ✓ Treatment does not define my future.
- ✓ Machines do not determine my destiny.
- ✓ I cooperate with medical wisdom, but I depend fully on divine power.
- ✓ Fear has no place in my body.
- ✓ Anxiety has no authority over my mind.
- ✓ I rest in the finished work of Christ.
- ✓ Healing is not something I must earn—it is something I receive.
- ✓ What Jesus finished, I do not question.
- ✓ What He completed, I do not delay.
- ✓ I declare progressive restoration, visible manifestation, and lasting health.
- ✓ I shall not die but live.
- ✓ I will testify of the Lord's faithfulness.
- ✓ My body aligns with heaven's verdict.
- ✓ It is finished—and I receive what is finished.

These declarations are not a denial of medical care, but a declaration of spiritual truth. We honor doctors, treatment, and wisdom—while placing our ultimate trust in the completed work of Christ.

Closing Declaration

I declare that the finished work of the Cross is active in my body now.
What Jesus completed, I receive.
What He bore, I refuse to carry.
By His stripes, I am healed—already.
I do not negotiate with symptoms. I do not argue with feelings.
I agree with the Cross. I speak from the Cross.
I do not speak from fear. I do not speak from symptoms.
What Jesus finished, I receive. What He purchased, I walk in.
What He declared complete, I will not call unfinished.

Final Chapter & Conclusion
"It Is Finished – Now Live Healed"

The final words Jesus spoke on the cross were not a cry of defeat. They were not a whisper of exhaustion. They were a declaration—clear, intentional, and complete.

"It is finished" (John 19:30).

That sentence did not mean His suffering was over; it meant the work was done. Redemption was secured. Sin was judged. Separation was bridged. And everything humanity would ever need to be restored to God—spirit, soul, and body—was fully paid for.

Nothing remained pending.

When Jesus said, *"It is finished,"* He was not speaking poetically. He was announcing a legal reality. In the original language, the phrase carried the meaning of *paid in full.* Not partially covered. Not awaiting future installments. Finished.

For many believers, healing still feels like something they are chasing rather than something they are standing on. They pray, they wait, they hope—but deep down, they wonder if the answer is still undecided. This chapter exists to settle that question once and for all.

- ✓ *Healing is not future.*
- ✓ *Healing is not conditional.*
- ✓ *Healing is finished.*
- ✓ *The Cross Already Spoke*

The cross was not only about forgiveness of sins; it was about restoration of life. Isaiah prophesied it centuries earlier when he wrote, "By His stripes we are healed" (Isaiah 53:5).

Notice the tense. Even before the cross, God spoke of healing as a certainty. Peter echoed the same truth after the resurrection, saying,
"By whose stripes ye were healed" (1 Peter 2:24).
Healed—not *will be*, not *might be*, but *were*.
The cross settled heaven's position on sickness forever. God did not leave healing undecided. He did not leave it dependent on human perfection or spiritual performance. He placed it squarely within the finished work of Christ.
That is why Paul could confidently declare,
"In all these things we are more than conquerors through Him that loved us" (Romans 8:37).
Not someday.
Not after everything feels better.
In all these things—right in the middle of real life.

Old Testament Foreshadowing: The Passover Night
Long before the cross, God painted a picture of complete redemption in Egypt. On the night of the Passover, the Israelites applied the blood of the lamb to their doorposts. Judgment passed over them, not because they were perfect, but because the blood was present.
Psalm 105 tells us something remarkable about that night: *"There was not one feeble person among their tribes."*
They left Egypt forgiven, protected, and strengthened. Redemption included physical restoration. God did not rescue them spiritually and abandon them physically. He never has.
The cross was the greater Passover. What the blood did on doorposts then, it does in hearts now—completely.

New Testament Reality: Living From Completion

After the resurrection, the apostles never preached healing as a distant possibility. They proclaimed it as a present reality. In Acts 3, Peter did not ask God if He was willing to heal the lame man at the gate called Beautiful. He declared what had already been authorized.

"Such as I have give I thee: In the name of Jesus Christ of Nazareth rise up and walk."

Peter wasn't begging heaven. He was enforcing what heaven had already decided.

A Modern Story: Learning to Stop Waiting

Daniel had loved God for years. He prayed faithfully and believed sincerely, but chronic migraines had followed him most of his adult life. He often said, *"I know God can heal me—when the time is right."*

One evening, while reading the Gospel of John, Daniel paused at the words, *It is finished*. For the first time, he realized something quietly unsettling: if it was finished then, what exactly was he waiting for now?

His prayers changed—not in volume, but in posture. He stopped asking God to do something new and began thanking Him for what was already done. When pain came, Daniel didn't panic or pretend it wasn't there. He simply reminded himself, *This doesn't change the truth.*

Over time, the migraines lost their authority. But more importantly, fear lost its grip. Daniel learned to live from rest instead of striving.

Heaven Is Already Settled

Jesus taught us to pray,

"Thy will be done in earth, as it is in heaven" (Matthew 6:10).

That prayer only works if heaven's will is already established. There is no sickness in heaven. No disease. No decay. No fear of relapse. Heaven is not debating healing.

Earth does not need a new decision from God. It needs alignment with what has already been decided.

Living Healed Does Not Mean Pretending

Living healed does not mean denying symptoms or rejecting wisdom. Faith is not fantasy. It does not shame the suffering or silence the hurting. Jesus never rebuked people for being sick—He rebuked storms, demons, and unbelief.

Living healed means anchoring your identity in truth even while walking through process. It means refusing condemnation when progress feels slow. It means trusting God's heart while using wisdom, medical help, and support without guilt.

A Gentle Invitation, Not a Demand

This book does not exist to pressure anyone. It does not condemn those still believing or suggest that suffering equals failure. It does not deny the value of doctors, medicine, or time. And it certainly does not promote hype or emotional manipulation.

- ✓ *It simply invites.*
- ✓ *It invites believers to rest where Christ finished.*
- ✓ *It invites weary hearts to stop striving.*
- ✓ *It invites the sick to come without fear of blame.*

Jesus never said, "Figure it out."

He said, *"Come unto Me."*

Now, Live From What Is Finished

You are not waiting on God.

Heaven is not undecided.

The cross already spoke.

Healing is not something you chase—it is something you receive and walk out, day by day, grounded in grace.

So live healed—not arrogantly, not anxiously, but anchored.

Let faith be quiet confidence.

Let praise be steady gratitude.

Let your life become a testimony, not of perfection, but of trust.

Because *it is finished* does not mean the journey ends.

It means the foundation is unshakable.

About the Author
'GERARD ASSEY'

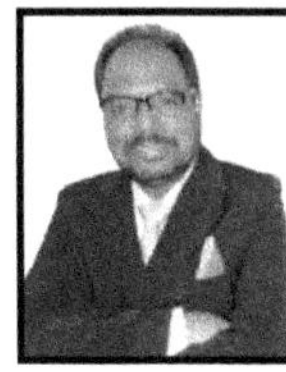

Gerard Assey is a Graduate in Economics, a PGD in Management (HRD) and holds a Doctorate in Leadership. Gerard holds several International Qualifications in Sales, Debt Collection, Training & Teaching, and is a 'Fellow' of the prestigious 'Institute of Sales & Marketing Management'-UK, a Certified NLP Practitioner, a 'Certified Trainer', an 'Accredited Management Teacher-Behavioral Sciences', a 'Certified Competency Facilitator', a 'Certified Management Consultant'- (the International credentials of a professional management consultant, awarded in accordance with global standards of the ICMCI); and a Certification from the University of Michigan in 'Successful Negotiation: Essential Strategies and Skills'

He is also a Member of the 'National Association of Sales Professionals' backed with several years experience in varied industries, both in India and Overseas. He also holds an 'Etiquette Consultant' Certification from the USA (by Sue Fox, Author of Best Seller: 'Business Etiquette for Dummies'. She has trained some of the top celebrities' world over). He was also a recipient of a scholarship for extensive training in Japan on 'Corporate Management for India'.

Gerard Assey is 'Founder & Chief Corporate Trainer' of the Group: '**Citius, Altius, Fortius Unlimited**'- an organization that **celebrated 20 years of Glorious Service** in 2021, focusing on 3 Core Competencies:

People. Performance. Profit; in functional areas of Sales & Marketing, HR & Organizational Development, covering Recruitment, Training & Consultancy!

Having managed organizations with large Sales Forces in India & Overseas, his specialization cover extensive areas of Sales Training (All levels - Presentation, Negotiation, Key/ Strategic Accounts Management & Managerial Skills for all sectors), Bid Proposal/ Capture Planning/ Management Trainings, Retail Sales, Customer Service & Customer Retention Programs, Training for Prevention & Collection of Debt, Self & Personal Development Programs (Time Management, Teamwork & Team Building, Business Etiquette & Personal Grooming, Leadership & Managerial Skills, People Management Skills, Train-the-Trainer etc), including preparation of Custom-designed Business Manuals for Internal (HR, Induction, and Sales etc) & External use (Instruction, User Manuals).

Gerard has successfully conducted over 6490 Trainings & Workshops (as of Dec '25) all across India, Middle East, Africa, Europe & S.E. Asia. Besides public programs conducted regularly, both in India & Overseas, he has some of the top names as clients whom he services from Single Owners to large Public & Government undertakings, covering all sectors, for their in-house needs.

His website: www.CollectionSkills.com is the only one in this part of the world to be featured in the 'Collections & Credit Risk Magazine-USA' under 'Who's Who in Training' and ranks TOP, along with other websites listed below on most search engines.

Gerard is author of 214 Books already (Jan 2026), all the books being available on all online platforms and outlets as E-books and Paperbacks

A few of our business related books:

1. Bite-sized Bits on Commonsense Management
2. Heart to Heart on Life's Principles'
3. How to become a Successful Manager
4. The Sales Professionals' Master Workbook of S.Y.S.T.E.M.S
5. The Professional Business Email Etiquette Handbook & Guide
6. The Professional Business Video-Conferencing Etiquette Handbook & Guide
7. Professional Presentation Skills
8. Exceptional Customer Service
9. Professional Tele-Marketing Skills
10. Professional Debt Collection Skills
11. The G.R.E.A.T. Sales & Service Workbook
12. Sales Training Advantage for Results (*The Ultimate Sales Training Manual to enable you stand out as a S.T.A.R.*)
13. CEO Daily Planner & Organizer
14. The Sales Professionals' Master Daily Planner
15. The Professional Debt Collector's Master Daily Planner
16. My Daily Planner & Organizer
17. MY EMERGENCY INFORMATION RECORD (Family Emergency & Peace of Mind Planner)
18. The Ultimate Therapist & Counselors Planner and Organizer
19. Building an Ethical Workplace
20. Managing Relationships at Work
21. Managing Business Meetings Effectively
22. Effective Delegation Skills
23. Goal Setting for Success
24. B2B Selling by Email
25. Professional Business Etiquette & Grooming
26. Dining Etiquette & Table Manners
27. Effective Networking Skills
28. Grooming, Etiquette & Manners for Teens, Young Adults & Future Leaders
29. Inter-Personal Skills
30. Get Ready, Get Hired!
31. Selling in a Recession
32. Effective Receivables Management in an Economic Downturn!
33. Real Estate & Property Sales Training
34. Credit Sales & Accounts Receivable Management

35. Selling Skills for Real Estate & Property Advisors
36. Take G.R.E.A.T. C.A.R.E!
37. Spa, Salon & Health Club Selling Skills
38. Selling Travel, Holiday & MICE Services
39. Selling Skills for Spa's, Salons & Health Clubs
40. Retailing in Salons & Spas
41. Selling Holiday, Vacation, Tours & Packages
42. The Power of Sales Referrals
43. Selling Luxury
44. Technical Selling Skills
45. Financial Advisors Sales Training
46. Dealing with Burnout at Work Monopolize Your Markets
47. Selling to Affluent Customers
48. Growing up with Grace
49. Financial Selling Skills
50. *The Effective Manager's Guide: Key Skills to Thrive*
51. From Aspiring to Inspiring: A Guide for New Managers on the Rise
52. The Power of Focus
53. Selling with Integrity: Sell Like Jesus The Perfect Role Model!
54. 31 Habits of Champions: Your 31-Day Journey to Greatness
55. Rejecting Grasshopper Talk: From Grasshopper to Giant-Killer-*Defeating Giants Daily!*
56. Navigate the AI-Powered Future of Bid & Proposals: Up-Skill to Stay Relevant with Alternative Career Paths & Opportunities
57. Hiring Sales Winners
58. Present with Impact
59. Success Unlocked: *Breaking Free from Habits that Hold You Back*
60. Complaints to Cheers, Feedback to Gold: Mastering Complaints Management
61. Thriving Together: *Cultivating Diversity, Equity, and Inclusion*
62. Coaching Skills for Sales Managers
63. Soaring to Success in Business & Leadership: Swifter, Higher, Stronger!
64. From Classroom to Podium: A Student's Guide to Powerful Public Speaking & Presentation Skills
65. Developing Self-Discipline
66. The CEO's 31-Day Power Plan: Unlocking Success through Essential Traits

67. Credibility Matters
68. A Winning Attitude
69. Bid & Proposal Management Using AI
70. Sales Forecasting: A Practical & Proven Guide to Strategic Sales Forecasting
71. Elevate & Energize: *50 Dynamic & Fun Activities for Peak Workplace Morale*
72. 'Sales SOS! Sales on Fire! *30 Days to Conquer Chaos & the Nightmares of Success!'*
73. Mastering Sales Managerial Skills: *Building High-Performing Teams & Driving Exceptional Results*
74. Eagle-Eyed Leadership: Unleashing the Power of 31 Lessons from Eagles
75. The Ultimate Employee Training Guide: *Training Today, Leading Tomorrow*
76. Being More Accountable at Work
77. Creating a Culture of Continuous Improvement
78. Effective Questioning & Listening Skills
79. The Power of Value Selling
80. The Growth Mindset
81. Mastering Professional Help Desk Skills
82. The Power to Lead with Empathy
83. Being Prepared: The Key to Unlocking Success
84. Youthful Spark-Youth Energizers, Activities and Games-Igniting the Fun in Youth
85. Ignite your Motivation for Success
86. Elevate Your Executive Presence: *Your Roadmap to Executive Excellence*
87. Smart Decisions: *Mastering Problem Solving with Strategic Solutions for Business Success*
88. Strategic Planning: *Developing and Implementing Strategic Plans to Achieve Long-Term Business Goals*
89. The Power of Stay Interviews
90. Developing G.R.I.T.
91. Adaptability
92. Diagnosis- *A Key Skill for Leadership*
93. The Burnout-Proof Salesperson: *The Master Guide to Preventing Stress & Burnout-* Strategies for Thriving in Sales
94. Learning from Failure: *Keys to Success*
95. Customer Success Management
96. Overcoming the Killers of Motivation
97. The C-Suite Code: *Mastering Skills for Executive Excellence'*

98. Dealing with Difficult Customers
99. Unlocking Your Potential: Mastering the Top 20 Life Skills for a Brighter Future
100. Nurturing Tomorrow's Leaders: *Essential Soft Skills Every Child Must Learn*
101. Lively & Fun Party Games for Seniors & Elders
102. Role Playing for Sales Champions: From Practice to Performance
103. Fun and Exciting Party Games for Kids
104. Case Studies for Sales
105. Role-Playing for Unbeatable Customer Service
106. Case Studies in Customer Service
107. Case Studies in Winning Negotiations
108. Case Studies in Management & Leadership
109. Case Studies in Human Resources & Talent Management
110. CEO Success Blueprint: The Essential Toolkit for CEOs and C-Level Executives
111. The Salesperson's Self-Coaching Guide: *Master Your Own Self-Coaching Plan for Success*
112. Overcoming Procrastination: *Your Ultimate Guide to Stop Delaying and Start Living Your Best Life*
113. When True Colors Are Exposed: *The Journey to Unmasking Humanity*
114. Life-Changing Habits for Teens: Teen Success Blueprint for a Bright Future
115. Workplace Stress-Free: *Proven Strategies to Thrive at Work and Beyond*
116. Objection Overruled: *The Ultimate Guide to Turning 'No' into 'Yes'*
117. Building Strong Teams: *A Comprehensive Guide to Team Building*
118. Ethical & Moral Leadership in Business: *Eliminating Unethical Practices & Building a Culture of Trust & Integrity*
119. Rising Strong: Building Positive: High Self-Esteem for a Fulfilling Life-*A Practical Guide for Students, Employees, Leaders & Entrepreneurs*
120 The Cheerful Mindset: Cultivating a Joyful Outlook Everyday
121. Leading Through Crisis: Case Studies on Crisis Management
122. Selling Beyond the Algorithms

From the Ministry side, Gerard graduated in the very first batch of Charis Bible College-India & had for over 9 years served as a Part-time Faculty at Charis Bible College-Chennai (Andrew Wommack Ministries-Colorado, USA).
He also holds a Diploma in Worship (a subject closest to his heart) from the JSOW and is also a graduate of the Advanced Mentorship Program (AMP) and the Circle Of Ministerial Engagement (C.O.M.E.) of Prophet Jerome Fernando and a Spiritual Son of the Esteemed Prophet.
An accomplished author of several Secular & Christian Books, Gerard has been on the board of a few international organizations and boasts of being the SON of the MOST HIGH GOD: An ordinary guy following an extraordinary GOD!

...And some of his most recent Christian Books being:

1. A Bouquet of Praises for My KING
2. Christian Jokes for the Serious Religious' Folks!
3. Jesus Healed You!
4. Praise24Ever! (also in Tamil version)
5. The 5G Network of GOD
6. Building Faith over F.E.A.R- FACE EVERYTHING AND RISE with JESUS
7. Hebrew and Greek Praise and Worship Words
8. Godly Mothers' and Grandmothers' Bible Story time for Kids!
9. Miracles of Jesus in Pictures
10. Raise your Praise all 365 Days
11. Thanking GOD with an Attitude of Gratitude
12. Meditating on the Attributes of GOD
13. Puppet Scripts
14. Alcohol Ruins, JESUS Reforms, Renews & Restores!
15. Habakkuk 2:2 Christian Daily Journal, Planner & Organizer
16. ABC of GOD's Word for Handwriting Practice
17. Daily Bible Verse Handwriting Practice (Building Godly Character & Faith through Cursive Handwriting Practice!)
18. Guiding Light: Fun & Faith-Building Bible Activities for Children
19. Rejecting Grasshopper Talk: From Grasshopper to Giant-Killer-*Defeating Giants Daily!*
20. Teen Titans of Faith: *Building Courage, Determination & Christ-like-Esteem*
21. I AM Empowered: *Unleashing Divine Power with Positive Declarations*

22. Be A Solution Provider-*From Passion to Purpose: A Biblical Guide to Being the Answer to the World!*
23. Miracles of JESUS
24. Parables of Jesus for a Meaningful Life!
25. A Grateful Heart: Importance of Sharing Testimonies of GOD's Grace
26. Melodies of Worship to JESUS: 31 Songs of Praise & Worship From My Heart to HIS!
27. I AM SO BLESSED!
28. My Daily Cup of Energizer
29. 31 Leadership Lessons *from* Jesus- *The Supreme Leader*
30. Peace Amidst Storms: A Biblical Guide to Conquering S.T.R.E.S.S.
31. Rise Above: 20 Biblical Eagle Lessons for Life's Triumphs
32. Godly Goal Setting: *The FAITHFUL Blueprint for a Purpose-Driven Life*
33. The Profound Attributes of our Mighty GOD: Understanding the 10S's of the Almighty
34. Worship Now, Worship Forever: *A Journey from Earthly Praise to Eternal Glory*
35. Unceasing Praise & Worship: *365 Days to Worship the King*
36. The ROAR Within: *Living with Purpose and Authority through the Power of the Holy Spirit*
37. From Potential to Purpose: Unlocking and Multiplying Your Talents & Gifts for Kingdom Impact
38. Songs from the Heart: *Worshipping GOD in Your Own Tune & Melody*
39. Awakening Praise & Worship: Hebrew & Greek Words to Raise Your Praise
40. Sing a NEW Song to the LORD Everyday: *Daily Devotions of Praise & Worship to Lift Your Heart & Glorify HIS Name*
41. *The* A.R.O.M.A. of True Worship: *Creating Worship That Delights God*
42. Becoming A Kingdom Champion: *Embracing God's Call for a Life of Purpose & Victory*
43. The Busy Businessman's Daily Devotional: 366 Crisp Truths to Start Your Day Strong
44. The Teacher's Heart: *Daily Devotions for Educators*
45. Anchored! *A 31-Day Devotional for Students Facing Life's Challenges*
46. Suddenly! Unlocking Unorthodox Breakthroughs through Unusual Worship
47. Overcoming Adversity: *Lessons from the Bible for Modern*

Challenges

48. LORD, Don't do it without me
49. Kingdom Leadership: *Biblical Principles for Modern Leaders*
50. Heartprints of God- *Growing God's Way:* Daily Devotions for Kids to Shine Bright
51. Send Judah First: Let your Praises Go up First to See the Mighty Move of GOD
52. DIVINE MOMENTS: *Recognizing, Embracing, Preparing, and Walking into Life-Changing Encounters with God*
53. Be a Builder in the Kingdom: *The C.E.M.E.N.T. Guide to Creating a Lasting Legacy*
54. Unshakable: *Pillars of Godly Womanhood* (Pillars of Faith That Changed History)
55. Lead Like a Shepherd: *14 Essential Traits for Pastoral Excellence*
56. The Worship Leader's Arsenal: *Powerful Exhortations to Ignite Thanksgiving, Praise & Worship*
57. Women of UnShakable Faith: *31-Day Devotional for Strength, Purpose & Influence*
58. Called to Teach: *A Complete 10-Week Training Guide for Impactful VBS Teachers*
59. Strumming for the KING: Cowboy Songs of Faith & Fire
60. The Ultimate Youth Camp Playbook: *50 Bible-Centered Indoor Games to Engage, Equip, and Empower Teens*
61. Glad in HIS Presence: *David's Revelation of GOD's Love & Mercy*
62. The Spirit Behind the Sound: *52 Devotionals for Worship Teams*
63. THE COWBOY'S COMPASS: *Riding the Trail of Faith with Grit & Grace*
64. Worship as My Weapon: *Living Victoriously through the Power of Praise*
65. A Worshipper Always Wins*: Living a Life of Victorious Worship*
66. Worship That Leads to the Throne: *Practical Strategies for Worship Leaders to Inspire Their Team & Usher People into God's Presence*
67. Worship as Warfare: *Conquering through the Sound of Surrender*
68. Watchmen on the Walls: *A 31-Day Devotional for Worship Teams*
69. KINGDOM BUSINESS: *52 Biblical Principles for GODLY*

Leadership & Wise Decisions

70. From Evening to Morning: *Rediscovering GOD's Sacred Hours*
71. Waves of Glory: *Worship through Dance, Flags, Staff & Sound*
72. WORSHIP TEAM BUILDER: *Guiding Your Team from Formation to Fruitfulness*
73. The Worship Leader's Master Training Manual
74. Skits for the King: Children's Plays for Every Church Occasion
75. Unbreakable: Building Strong Marriages and Families God's Way *(From Vows to Victory)*
76. Songs for my King: *A 31-Day Journey of Praise*
77. Building Powerful Children: *Raising a Generation That Will Shape the Future for God*
78. Character Before Chords: *The Heart of the True Worshipper*
79. 365 Days Before His Throne: A Worshipper's Daily Declarations
80. Broken to Built: *How GOD Restores Lives, Heals Hearts & Uses Broken People for HIS Glory*
81. Fear Did Not Come from God: *Discerning the Source, Dismantling the Stronghold & Walking in Power, Love & a Sound Mind*
82. THE GOD OF BEGINNINGS: *Positioning Your Life for What God Is About to Start*
83. HEALED ALREADY: IT IS FINISHED! Receiving What the Cross Has Completed!

Besides regularly contributing to business & trade journals, including international ones such as the 'Creative Training Techniques' and the 'Sales News' of the U.S.A, He is also a member of several prestigious bodies & trade associations, having participated in many Conferences & Workshops in India & Overseas.

Prior to his last assignment of leading & managing a large MNC as head, Gerard had a 3-year stint in the Middle East as a Consultant with a leading British Consultancy Firm.

As the past ‘Official Country Representative’ for the International Business Award- ‘THE STEVIES’-(the business world’s own Oscar) for about 4 years- he ensured a few Indian companies that qualify for the same every year!

Gerard can be contacted at:

Email: training@Sales-Training.in,training@CollectionSkills.com
Websites:

www.Sales-Training.in
www.EtiquetteWorks.in
www.CollectionSkills.com
www.RetailSalesTraining.in
www.SalesTrainingIndia.com
www.ManualPreparation.com
www.TrainingWithPuppets.com
www.FirstContactAcademy.com
www.SalesAndMarketingRecruiter.com

www.ingramcontent.com/pod-product-compliance
Ingram Content Group UK Ltd.
Pitfield, Milton Keynes, MK11 3LW, UK
UKHW021340190726
13845UKWH00027B/654

9 788199 513495